C000246990

DISEASES

MOR

VENOSITY, VARICOCELE, HÆMORRHOIDS,
AND VARICOSE VEINS,

AND THEIR

TREATMENT BY MEDICINES.

BY

J. COMPTON BURNETT, M.D.,

*Author of "Natrum Muriaticum," "Gold as a
Remedy in Disease," "Fistula and its Radical
Cure by Medicines," "Diseases of the
Spleen," etc.*

FIFTH EDITION

B. Jain Publishers (P) Ltd.
USA — Europe — India

DISEASES OF THE VEINS

5th Impression: 2012

Published by Kuldeep Jain for
B. JAIN PUBLISHERS (P) LTD.
1921/10, Chuna Mandi, Paharganj, New Delhi 110 055 (INDIA)
Tel.: +91-11-4567 1000   Fax: +91-11-4567 1010
Email: info@bjain.com   Website: **www.bjain.com**

Printed in India by
J.J. Offset Printers

ISBN: 978-81-319-1793-0

PREFACE TO FOURTH EDITION.

———————

THE First Edition of this work was written nearly fifteen years ago ; since then many hundreds of cases of varicocele, hæmorrhoids, and varicose veins have passed under my observation and professional care. And are my views still the same in regard to the amenability of Diseases of the Veins to medicinal treatment ?

They are the same, and now stand amply confirmed.

To this Edition is added a "General Survey of Varicosis and Varicose Veins," and this will show the direction in which my clinical work has developed, *i.e.*, I now lay more stress on the diagnosis of the cause in each individual case, going first to the topographic relationships of its origin when obstructive, thence to the constitutional origin of the non-obstructive varieties, and finally to the therapeutic indications. In this manner the treatment becomes more methodical : first, we deal with the obstruction where such exists, and in these cases hæmorrhage is an unusual occurrence. Secondly, we proceed to cure the blood diseases where such exist, and here hæmorrhages are common and often severe ; when these blood diseases are cured the hæmorrhages cease, and then the vein-medicines proper and the anti-traumatics come into play

J. COMPTON BURNETT.

PREFACE TO SECOND AND THIRD EDITIONS.

A Second and a Third Edition of my "Diseases of the Veins" being called for, I have carefully revised it and added some new matter.

As to what I have ventured to call the *Venous Zigzag* on the thorax, I willingly admit Dr Edward Blake's claim to priority, he having called attention to the condition thereby expressed in a paper read by him at the Liverpool Congress ; at the same time the name is mine and the observation original to me.

PREFACE TO FIRST EDITION.

THIS little book is not a complete treatise on the pathology and therapeutics of diseases of the venous system, but comprehends merely my own experience (Part I.) in the MEDICINAL TREATMENT OF DILATED VEINS in various regions of the body.

Nevertheless, it is hoped that some few practical hints herein contained will be of interest and clinical value to others who may wander the same way, and to make it more useful to such, the Second Part contains indications for about 50 remedies likely to be useful in varicose conditions.

The more I learn of practical medicine, the more I am impressed with the wise words of *Fernelius* . . . *Nulla usquam est remediorum penuria, sed nostra eorum plerumque turpis ignoratio.* Verily, remedies are a great deal more than mere "aids to faith in the weary time."

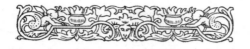

The Medicinal Treatment
of
Diseases of the Veins.

GENERAL SURVEY OF VARICOSIS AND VARICOSE VEINS.

VARICOSE veins may owe their dilated state either to (1), a blood disease; (2), to weak vein walls or valves; (3), to a mechanical obstruction to the flow of the blood heartwards; (4), heart disease; or (5), it may be part and parcel of what might be called the *"ptosic"* constitution.

2

Where the origin is merely due to (3) topic obstruction, the best plan is to find out the obstruction and remove it, and then the veins return, more or less, to their proper size ; and there then only remains a loss of tone in the vein walls ; here such remedies as *Arnica*, *Bellis*, *Ferrum*, *Pulsatilla*, and *Hamamelis* will suffice to finish the cure. Where the obstruction cannot be found, or having been found cannot be removed, *Fluoric acid* has most frequently helped me.

But the obstruction can very frequently be found and remedied radically, and then a very beautiful cure is the end result of the treatment.

How to understand Varicosis from Obstruction

If we dam up a given river at a certain place, all the little streams and rivulets that debouch into it *above the dam* will fill up and swell in volume, and very likely overflow their banks and flood the environs. Now, if we want to get rid of this overflow of the banks, we may certainly raise the banks and so hem in the water, but in this way we increase the volume of the rivulets, and the heightened banks need much and constant attention ; but if we go down to the dam and remove it, we have no further difficulty with the streams and rivulets, for they will run on and empty themselves into the river, just as the latter will run on into the sea.

Now so it is with varicose veins from obstruction; the obstruction is the dam that prevents the smaller veins from duly emptying themselves into the larger ones. We may, to continue our simile, heighten the banks by putting on elastic stockings, but the better plan is to go down to the obstructive dam and remove it, for just as the rivulets with the higher banks increase in volume, so do varicose veins that are merely held in by mechanical support.

The support afforded by bandages and elastic stockings to the varicose veins has no other effect than such support: the ailment goes on developing just the same, and, as a matter of fact, the support often does much harm. Let me explain. As I have already made use of the damming up of the river to illustrate the nature of obstructive varicosis, so the same simile will serve to show the ultimate and further effects of elastic stockings or other support, viz. :—

1. Dam up a river and all its above-dam tributaries will increase in volume until the dam is overcome, or until the volume of water in the river reaches the level of the top of the dam.

2. If the dam is strong enough and high enough, the beds of the said tributaries will presently no

longer suffice for the volume of
water contained in them, and the
banks of the tributary streams will
overflow : now here, if we raise and
strengthen these banks, we merely
remove the overflow further up
stream, and the feeders of the
tributaries will in their turn increase
in volume and overflow *their* banks,
—*i.e.*, the increase in volume of the
water dammed up is extended
further up stream, it is not got rid
of. So it is with the elastic stocking or bandage ; it gets rid of no
varicosis, but removes the influence
of the obstruction further up heartwards, just as the heightened and
strengthened above-dam banks
remove the danger of overflow
further up stream. Of course, this

may under circumstances be a good
thing to do, but such is its limita-
tion.

Hence in every case of varicosis
I am in the habit of first trying to
find out the mechanical cause of the
varicosis. Above the level of the
heart we do not often meet with
varicose veins, because gravitation
is sufficient to overcome any
moderate obstruction. Below the
diaphragm, on the other hand,
varicose veins are very common,
because here gravitation tends to
increase any tendency to varicosis.

A swelled or enlarged liver is a
frequent cause of varicose veins of
the right leg; a swelled spleen has
a similar effect on the venous circulation of the left lower extremity.

Constipation has a like effect on either lower extremity, according to where the accumulated fæces lie. In ladies, uterine enlargement and displacement act similarly. One-sided varicosis is often caused by ovarian enlargements. Thus, I was once consulted for a young lady whose left lower extremity was the seat of very severe varicosis: the veins were so badly dilated that the limb had a hideous aspect,—so much so that all idea of marriage had been given up; the well-fitting stocking certainly supported the veins, but otherwise only tended to render the whole limb varicosic. I readily ascertained the location of the dam or obstructive element in the case, viz., there was a consider-

able enlargement of the left ovary,
with severe concomitant leucorrhœa.
This ovarian enlargement appeared
to me to be due to chronic inflammation of a sycotic nature.   I set to
work with antisycotics, and in a few
months the enlargement lessened,
and finally disappeared entirely; and
in proportion as the enlargement
lessened so the varicosis likewise
diminished, and also the leucorrhœa,
and finally the varicose veins could
no longer be found. The young lady
re-appeared in society, and she
presently married and had her first
baby last year.

Less than two years ago a Com-
mander in the Royal Navy, a very
healthy, well-preserved man, about

forty years of age, consulted me
in regard to an enormous varix
of the right groin as big as a small
orange, and the thing was all the
more alarming as the wall of the
varix had become thin, and being
in the bend of the groin, mechanical
support was practically impossible,
so of course it appeared that patient
would have to quit the service.
There being no heart affection, no
blood disease, no primary vein
disease and no history of any local
lesion or disease of any sort, I
made a careful examination of the
abdominal organs, and could only
make out a not very considerable
enlargement of the left lobe of the
liver. I therefore set about curing
the liver, though I did not think

the said enlargement sufficient to
account for such an enormous varix.
However, as soon as the liver had
been brought back to the normal,
the varix was reduced to a mere
nothing, and in a few months the
delighted patient hastened off on
active service, looking forward to
becoming in due course an Admiral.

The remedies which cured this
case were *Carduus Mariæ θ*, *Chelidonium majus θ*, and *Chelone glabra
θ*. For an account of the two
former remedies see my "Greater
Diseases of the Liver." and my
"Diseases of the Spleen and their
Remedies" respectively. As to the
last-named remedy—*Chelone glabra*
—I should like to say that its *seat* of
action is the left lobe of the liver,

and it *line of action* is in the direction of the navel, bladder, and uterus, while the "line of action" of *Carduus* is horizontal from liver to spleen, or conversely. At the first blush this looks fanciful, but the competent can readily verify it clinically.

Where the varicosis of the lower extremities preponderates on one side, but is present in both, it is useful to trace the history of the origin of the varices, and find out where it began and how it developed, and thus a diagnosis of the dam, if any, is greatly facilitated.

Where the lower extremities are both equally involved, and the hypogastric veins are also dilated, it is often due to indurated abdominal glands. Thus several years since a city merchant consulted me for such a state, he being desirous of getting married. Almost all the superficial veins of the extremites were dilated, and also the hypegastric veins ; the largest varicose veins were about the size of goose quills, the smaller ones about that of crow quills, so the aspect was ugly indeed. After about two years' treatment the veins were reduced about three-fourths, and the marriage has now been fixed for the near future.

I was led to diagnose indurated abdominal glands, from the visible and feelable hypertrophy and induration of his inguinal glands, which were cleary inherited and not acquired.   Nosodes   were the chief remedies.

The diagnosis of the seat of the dam is of very great importance in these cases.   Where one lower extremity is enlarged from per turbed circulation in the deep-lying veins of the limbs, looking like phlegmasia alba dolens, but occur-ring in the male, and not necessarily with any increase of sensation—the left leg is most commonly involved— the condition would appear to bear some relationship to the spleen, and may, perhaps, be to the spleen what myxœdema is to the thyroid.

Thus, a gentleman consulted me early in the current year (1894) for a considerable enlargement of the left leg, in aspect very much like

the ordinary white leg. He was
also suffering from scarring acne,
and the skin of his face was very
shiny. The spleen was notably
enlarged. Patient dated the swelling of the leg to an attack of
mountain fever which he had four
years ago in Colorado, since when
his enlargement had existed. He
had had gonorrhœa years ago, and
had also been twice vaccinated.
Vaccination at times, perhaps always, causes a certain amount of
tumefaction of the spleen, as does
also gonorrhœa, and I have over
and over again seen varicosis follow
common gonorrhœa ; examples of
this I could cite in numbers.

Urtica urens θ in small material
doses greatly lessened the enlarge-

ment of the leg in a few weeks. I cite this case thus quite shortly, to exemplify the usefulness of diagnosing the dam in cases of obstructive varicosis.

HÆMORRHOIDS.

Hæmorrhoids are essentially varicose veins of the anus and rectum. Here the first point to elucidate in each new case is the place of the dam—a not always easy task—but the anal region is very apt to harbour piles of obstructive origin, but which at the same time have become a substantive disease, and the vicarious outlet for the divers constitutional taints to which man is liable.

There is no such a thing as primary piles,—they are all either hypostatico-obstructive or merely obstructive, or from pressure from above, or from constitutional ailments, which, all lumped together, constitute the hæmorrhoidal diathesis, notably of German authors.

The frequent hæmorrhages from the hæmorrhoids are, in my judgment, all of constitutional origin, and constitutional treatment will cure such, but the *constitutional cause* must be got rid of before a radical cure can be effected either of the hæmorrhoids or of the hæmorrhoidal bleedings. To stop the bleeding by operation on the veins or on the part, is a proceeding that, in my judgment, should land the

3

operator into a medical court of inquiry. And quelling the bleeding with remedies without regard to the constitutional cause or causes, is not infrequently followed by constitutional disaster : anal bleedings are very often disease-outflows.

Now let any one of ordinary common-sense and understanding, whether medical or lay, tell me— How can it be seriously maintained that diseases of the veins are to be dealt with by surgery ? The surgical aid in vein affections only comes in as a last resort where nothing else can be done, and even then it is but a sorry uncertain old crutch.

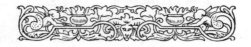

PART 1.

WHEN a man comes forward with a proposition not generally received by his fellows in his own walk of life, it behoves him to proceed inductively and independently. If he does this he is proceeding scientifically, and trained minds, not being overladen with prejudice, soon know where they are in dealing with his proposition. Experience proves that a proposition may be demonstrably true, and that it may yet meet with only a very limited acceptance; especially is this the case with new truths, and truths that involve unpleasant consequences. And when a person has once committed himself, once taken sides, he is very apt to go on thenceforth for ever —for *his* ever—from the standpoint of a *parti pris.*

Most medical men are pretty well agreed that Diseases of the Veins are not amenable to drug treatment in any important degree. I refer more especially to general varicosis, hæmorrhoids, varicocele, and varicose veins. These affections are therefore relegated to the domain of the surgeon ; and, no doubt, the surgery of the veins —particularly of hæmorrhoids—is now nearly perfect, being nearly bloodless and painless. That is very beautiful, and a matter of

sincere congratulation for us all.
It being pretty well perfect, the
question may not unreasonably be
raised . . . Is *surgery,* then, the
ONLY crutch to rely upon; has medicine *nothing* to say to the behoof
of healing affections of the veins ?

May not venous subjects fairly
say to the *physicians*—What have
you all been doing the past two
thousand years ; have you not, with
all your learning, vivisections and
mortisections, poisonings and drug-
provings, and your never-ending
ransacking of all creation for new
remedies ; have you not herewithal
been able to hit upon some gentle
innocuous means of bringing back
a few dilated veins to their normal
calibre ?

And would they be so *very* far
wrong, if, individually, they were to
continue in some such a strain as
this . . . What use is it to me,
with my baggy veins, that you dub
them with big names and learnedly
talk about hæmorrhoids, with hypertrophy of surrounding connective
tissue, varicocele, varicose veins,
varicosis, and all that, if I am *merely*
an object of study for you, and my
miseries only so many classes and
sub-classes in your nosological natural history ; and, having duly and
scientifically classified my peccant
parts, you bow me out with a
placebo, and show me thereafter
the way to the amphitheatre ?

But, then, this is not a thinking
age for the many ; only a few, in

the present hurry and flurry, and race after riches, can find time to go after "a more excellent way."

Oddly enough, the *art of healing*, pure and simple, is not in great repute nowadays ; indeed, it is almost a reproach to fling one's self body and soul into the business of healing, and herein try to do better than one's father did. Nay, it is even dangerous for a man of good repute to strike out a new path in therapeutics, and *try* to cure what 'the solid phalanx of and ancient trades union has ever held to be incurable ; if he do, he will infallibly be looked at askance, and no one will thank him, while many will seek to deride and vilify him. The reason of this lies

largely in the history of medicine
and of mankind ; bad ware has
been so often brought forward as
good that no one may be much
blamed for looking with some sus-
picion on all new notions.

Now, I am coming forward with
the thesis that atonic dilated veins
may, in many instances, be made to
shrink to their original size by the
proper use of medicines, administered internally and aided by certain
auxiliaries,—in other words, varicosis, hæmorrhoids, varicocele and
varices are amenable to drug-treat-
ment, and therefore surgery, in this
department of diseases of the veins,
is to be superseded by medicines.
Surgeons will no doubt object to
being thus ousted, and will probably

not fail to vent their wrath upon me. Good, my ireful brethren, you have done that before in another subject,* and yet truth is gaining thereby, and a certain step in advance has been made.

Of course you will perceive that neither there, nor here, am I originating anything ; I have merely been sitting at the feet of Hahnemann, and have come out to do battle for this great truth.

In the sincere hope that some truth-loving and truth-seeking brother may read this, and be desirous of seeking the path I have wandered, I will give it step by step, just as I have come. It is an honourable

---

* *"Curability of Cataract with Medicines."*

path, wherein walk many good men and true, who are striving to make the physician's business one of *healing the sick, cito, tuto, et jucunde* ; the path is not easy to travel, neither is it always daylight therein, but it has just one safe and sure hand-railing running along it from end to end, and that is . . . the LAW OF SIMILARS. There are other guides, but they do not go all the way ; they are only here and there, so we will, in the following pages, just hold on to . . . LIKE CURES LIKE. We are the more constrained to do so as we know no other safe guide in therapeutics.

The surgical treatment of diseases of the veins may be reduced

to three fundamental parts, viz.—
Local astringents ; pressure, by way
of support ; and the so-called radical
operations with the knife, or its
equivalent.

GENERAL VARICOSIS eludes the
surgeon entirely, for surgery must
necessarily be only local. But when
we have to deal with such local manifestations of varicosis or venosity,
the scholastic physician forthwith
hands over the case to the surgeon
for operation or for surgical appliances. Thus with HÆMORRHOIDS :
The physician gives his aperients,
with perhaps a local astringent, and
gradually the state of things gets
worse, and then the patient learns
that there is nothing for it but a
surgical operation. What a terrible

prospect, even in these days of
perfect anæsthetic and antiseptic
surgery ! Apart from the ultimate
effects of shock—a thing no one
seems to take cognizance of—
cutting off the piles cannot,
as a rule, reasonably be called
curing. And this shock to the
whole economy, arising from an
operation for piles, tells its tale
for many a year afterwards—
indeed, the sufferer often never
recovers from it entirely. If
we follow Hahnemann's method
of historical case-taking we see
strange things, as to the really
primitive causes of diseases. In my
own practical experience I trace
cases of diabetes and cataract to
the surgical traumatism inflicted in

operating for piles. But more of this anon.

Again, with VARICOCELE : This is held to be entirely within the surgeon's domain. I well remember the first case I ever saw was in one of the clinics in the Vienna General Hospital. It was an exquisite case, and the subject an individual of about 25, suffering really from general varicosis, but this condition was most pronounced in the spermatic veins from evident causes. Our genial and much-beloved teacher said to us . . . "There is nothing for it, gentlemen, but the radical cure." I inquired what the "radical cure" was, and learned, of course, that it meant a surgical operation. That is still the orthodox teaching, but it is as false as it is cruel, and as shallow as it is false. A *merely* surgical cure is no *real* cure at all, and in its very nature cannot be radical ; better than nothing, no doubt, and often nearly as good as a cure, but still not a healing, in its true sense.

Finally, with VARICOSE VEINS : The scholastic physician has here nothing whatever to say, beyond recommending his own favourite *elastic stocking* maker. The surgeon comes in to treat any hæmorrhage that may eventually occur from a ruptured vein, or to treat the varicose ulcers and bad legs. All mere patch-work and cobbling, if nothing more be done.

But if we are to relegate the simple surgical treatment of vein diseases to the lumber-room, what is to take its place ? The answer is . . . *Scientific medicinal treatment,* and in therapeutics that means specific constitutional (homœopathic) treatment ; for science in therapeutics and homœopathy are synonymous terms.

The first time I became aware of the fact that the veins could be specifically affected with medicines at all, was in reading a book by Dr. Richard Hughes, entitled "A Manual of Pharmacodynamics," that was a new revelation to me in so many ways. It has been called "Homœopathic Milk for Allopathic

Babes ;" it would be a good thing
for the world if the allopaths would
but partake freely of this precious
milk. However, there is one condition absolutely necessary to its
digestibility, viz., the allopathic
babe must have a clean tongue,
and a stomach that calls loudly for
healthy therapeutic food, or it will
disagree with him. For, if his
tongue be coated with crass prejudice, and his stomach gorged with
medical conventionalism and scho-
lasticism, he will be unable to take
it up or assimilate it. And if he
cannot bear the milk, how is he to
partake of the more solid food of
the Organon. Well, the special
article I refer to is that on *Acidum
fluoricum*, which to me, then, was

an altogether new and unheard-of *remedy.* The part that so impressed me runs thus :—

"Under its use whitlows have been blighted ; fistulæ—lachrymal and dental —have healed ; *varicose veins have shrunk to half their size ;* fresh hair has grown on a bald head, and moist palms have regained their healthy dryness."

This was good seed sowed, and it has borne much good therapeutic fruit in my subsequent professional life. An exquisite case of *Alopecia areata* recovered so completely, under the prolonged use of *Acidum fluoricum,* that a long-worn wig could be put off. This was observed by me while house-surgeon at the Hardman Street Homœopathic Dispensary in Liverpool ; and it was

4

there, too, that I first had an opportunity of testing this remarkably bold assertion of Dr Hughes, namely, that varicose veins would shrink to half their size under the influence of fluoric acid.

THE LAMP-LIGHTER'S CASE OF EXCESSIVE VARICOSITY OF THE LEFT INTERNAL SAPHENOUS VEIN.

A middle-aged man, by occupation a lamp-lighter, came under observation at the Dispensary for an enormously dilated vein of the left thigh. At its highest and largest end, just where it dips down to the femoral vein through the saphenous opening of the *fascia lata*, it was as large as a child's wrist ;

and near the knee, about the size of a man's little finger, so that there was no inconsiderable danger of its rupturing and causing dangerous hemorrhage. It was not the local expression of general varicosis, but arose from a mechanical obstruction in this wise : Patient had sowed his wild oats lang syne, and as part of the harvest had reaped a big bubo in the left groin. This had sloughed, and been burned with a strong acid, and there resulted as scar, a cicatricial surface of the size of a man's palm, and this scar-tissue in contracting had very much narrowed the entrance of the long saphenous vein, through the opening of the *fascia lata* into the deeper-lying crural vein. Then, in those days, lamp-lighters used to do their work with the aid of light ladders, and were in the habit of sliding down them scores of times a day, and thus the vein, that had become dilated from the lateral pressure of the venous blood, coursing up the saphena, having such a contracted entrance, became still more disturbed in its function ; hence the enormous dilatation.

Patient received *Acidum fluoricum* 6 in pilules, and was directed to take one four times a day, and come and report himself every fortnight till further orders. This he did for several months, with the result that the enormously dilated vein shrank to about one-third of its original size, and this notwith-

standing patient's continuance at
his usual occupation. No auxiliaries and no local applications or
appliances were used, and the diet
was not altered. When I saw him
last the varicosis had ceased to be
of any inconvenience ; it was no
longer dangerous in anythings like
the same degree, as the vein felt
firm and strong. Considering the
irremediable mechanical hindrance
at its inlet, the result seemed to me
so striking *that I have ever since
gone in very strongly for the medicinal treatment of varicosis under
all circumstances*, and the satisfaction one has in such medicinal
treatment is truly great.

*   *   *   *

It is not medically orthodox
to believe in the amenability of
Diseases of the Veins to drug
treatment, and my own medical
education having been ultra-ortho-
dox, I thought it would be only
fit that I should show what led me
away from the generally received
notions in this regard. This I
have done in the foregoing, and the
question may now be fairly put to
any candid medical mind . . . If a
greatly dilated, long saphenous
vein, whose inlet was considerably
narrowed, could be so materially
modified in its physiological life
by internal drug treatment alone
— *the mechanical hindrance at the
inlet still remaining*—is it not at
least probable that many other

forms of varicosis would likewise
yield to properly chosen remedies ?
That such is the case I shall now
proceed to shew, Before doing so,
however, it might not be amiss to
state that this notion has not originated with me or with Dr Hughes ;
this genial writer was my immediate
devencier, and until I read his article
on *Acidum fluoruum*, I had never
even heard that any one ever at-
tempted the medicinal cure of
varices. Since then I have, of
course, become fully aware that
the thing dates back to Hahnemann and others, and that *capable*
homœopaths have herein followed
in his wake for a good half-century ;
careless homœopaths, however, often
decline the bother and trouble con-

sequent upon the acceptance of the
dogma that vein diseases may be
cured with medicines, more especially since the surgery has become
almost painless by reason of the
anæsthetics, and bloodless by means
of the neat, elegant, and effective
surgical proceedings at the operations ; more particularly is this the
case with piles. Yet, even here,
how much is a kindly, gentle,
medicinal cure to be preferred !
Far be it from me to detract from
and honour due to my surgical
brethren ; nay, I am free to admit
that, had my hand possessed the
chirurgical cunning that lies in
theirs, I should no doubt have
also suffered from the surgeon's
itch, and I may never have had

the *patience* to try medicines as I have done, in the very worst forms of piles and other varicoses, and thus finally triumphed, to my own intense satisfaction.

Necessitas non habet legem, and, moreover, she is the lawful mother of invention, as we have it in our own vernacular. While giving, therefore, all due honour to surgery, I must call very special attention to what may be termed . . .

CHRONIC CHIRURGICAL TRAUMATISM.

As far as I am aware, I have never read anything about this very important subject in any books ; what I think I know thereon has been read in Natures ever-open book, that comes to us page by page, word by word, and letter by letter, in the form of living human beings that are technically termed patients. I am not referring to ordinary traumatism, nor yet to surgical shock, but to the chronic traumatism that is caused by the surgical operation *per se*—here for piles more particularly—and which gives an impression to the organism that becomes chronic, and whose effects are seen years and years thereafter. And I do not think the traumatism is one whit the less for the anæsthetics, so that whether a patient *feels* any pain at the operation or not, is, in the present sense, quite a matter of indifference.

I could offer a good many proofs of this proposition did space allow, but let us at least think over the matter a little. To begin with traumastism is *admitted* when it arises from *contre-temps* in obstetric practice, and no one of experience will be disposed to deny it when ascribed to blows, falls, railway accidents, and the like. This is so well recognised in homœopathic practice that many successful cures have been wrought by falling back on the traumatic etiology of, may be, twenty or more years ago.

What made me *first* think about it was the very frequent observation, in taking the cases of

cataract* patients, that *operations
for piles* were so often a part of
their life history. It could not be
accident or mere coincidence, I
thought ; if *mere* coincidence, it is,
to my mind, very strange.

Thus I am at present treating a
patient for *diabetes mellitus*, and the
whole of her almost hopeless case—
she is a veritable sugar-maker *en
gros*—points unmistakably to the
traumatic origin of her complaint,
the trauma being an operation for
piles.

Ophthalmologists are in no
doubt about cataract being often
due to blows and injuries ; indeed,

---

* Operation for cataract has been known
to be soon followed by complete loss of
speech and memory.

traumatic cataract is a recognised variety of that distressing affection. When we consider the exquisite sensitiveness of the rectum, and its extreme tenderness and resentfulness of foreign interference ; when we remember the hyperæsthesia of the parts in a *bad* case of piles—let sufferers from piles say whether the rectum is a sensitive part !—there is, to say the least, nothing against the hypothesis that an operation for piles may, and does, make an abiding impression upon the organism that may years thereafter culminate in serious organic mischief. Still, I have not arrived at this conclusion from *a priori* reasoning, but induce it from observation in actual cases.

We need not enter into the matter any further here, as we are now concerned with the medicinal treatment of diseases of the veins, and to follow out the subject of *chronic chirurgical traumatism* would be digressive ; I merely mention it parenthetically, as it were, and commend it to the consideration of those whose refuge is the knife.

GENERAL
CONSTITUTIONAL VENOSITY.

There are certain subjects whose venous systems are exceedingly prone to ail ; if they have anything wrong with their hearts, it is pretty sure to be the venous side of it ; if they get dyspepsia, it arises from congestion of the ' portal system of

veins ; if they suffer from headaches, it is from venous stasis ; if
they get constipated, piles develop
at once ; if they stand much, or
wear a tight garter, they get varices
of the legs ; if the *uro-genetic* system
gets irritated or injured, and fails
to get tone-giving natural relief,
they have varicocele, or menstrual
troubles from dilated veins of the
ovaries and broad ligaments, as the
case may be. They are *constitu-
tionally venous,* and suffer from
passive congestions at all turns.
Such a one was the following :—

CASE OF GENERAL VARICOSIS, VARICOCELE, AND VARICOSE VEINS.

A gentleman, about thirty years
of age, came under my observation

on October 17, suffering from chronic prostatitis, varicocele, and varicose ulcers of the legs. At a glance one could see that he was a venous subject ; as he was swarthy, pensive, and melancholy, and had long slender limbs. Almost every region of his venous circulation showed signs of dilatation, having an enormous left-sided varicocele, and very pronounced baggy varices of the legs. His internal saphenous veins were like big ropes. Around his left ankle were varicose ulcers, and the whole neighbourhood around was very dark, almost black in places. He stated that this left ankle had been in this state nearly all his life. General health fairly good, except some lack of virility, but bandaging his legs was, of course, burdensome, and the varicocele was very inconvenient, more especially in view of approaching marriage.

℞ *Ferrum Phosphoricum*, 6 trituration ʒiv. To take four grains in water three times a day.

Nov. 12. The spermatic veins are not any smaller, as far as he can perceive ; the veins in his lower extremities *are* smaller ; *and the dark places under the left ankle are turning to a proper flesh colour.*

Repeat the same remedy.

Dec. 8. The varicocele is much smaller—"At one time its existence was very inconvenient ; now I hardly notice it," said he. The varicose ulcers have healed up, and the skin around is assuming a healthy hue.

Repeat.

Jan. 8. Has had gatherings in the place where the black patch *was*. All the varicose veins and varicocele *much* better.

℞ *Kali. Chlor.*, 6 trit., ℨiv. Four grains in water three times a day.

April 14. The veins are all getting smaller ; the foot has *completely* healed (had had it nearly all his life !) The varicocele very much better, and also the varices of the lower extremities, the *venae saphenae longae* having notably diminished in size. These few months of treatment have wrought a great change

in the patient and in the *man,* and
I accordingly gave him permission
to get married. He is, of course,
not yet *completely* cured of his
general varicosis,—the time has
been to short for that,—but the
improvement is so great that
all obvious unsightliness has disappeared, and this is no small
boon to a man contemplating
marriage.

This case has given me great
satisfaction, as a worse one has
never come under my observation
in a man of that age. I made use
of no local application whatever ;
neither was any change made either
in his diet, mode of life (standing
nearly all day), or place of abode,
but he continued the bandage to

his foot, to which he had been accustomed for more than twenty years.

He tells me his father suffered similarly. Practical men will agree with me that it is not very usual to have trouble from varicose veins at ten years of age, as this gentle-man had, and that, as it went on without getting any better for twenty years, the present remark-able amelioration is, and can be, due to nothing else but the medicines ; and this being so—and considered in conjunction with the lamplighter's case—*my present thesis, that venous dilatation can be cured or amelior-ated by medicines*, is established. The basis on which it is established is narrow, perhaps, and therefore we will proceed to widen it, by citing other evidence in its favour.

Before doing so, however, let me be allowed to give what surgery has to say on varicocele. I will quote from a young promising surgeon, of the very latest date. In the *Lancet* of July 17, 1880, we read ;—

PART OF A CLINICAL LECTURE ON THE RADICAL CURE OF VARICOCELE BY THE GALVANIC ECRASEUR, DELIVERED AT THE WESTMINSTER HOSPITAL ON JULY 3RD, 1880, BY A. PEARCE GOULD, M.S., F.R.C.S., ASSISTANT-SURGEON TO THE HOSPITAL, AND LECTURER ON ANATOMY TO THE MEDICAL SCHOOL.

GENTLEMEN,—Although there are very many cases of vaicocele in which no treatment, or only palliative measures, are required, you will meet with others in which it will be your duty to undertake the permanent or radical cure of the varix. These cases are as follow :—1. Where the testicle is atrophying. 2. Where the varicocele is double, especially if an examination of the semen shows an absence of spermatozoa, or the patient, being married, is sterile. 3. Where the opposite testicle is lost or useless from tumour, orchitis, epididymitis, or injury. 4. Where the varix is large and increasing, in spite of palliative treatment. 5. Where the varix causes much pain, or interferes with proper exercise and necessary work. 6. Where it is the occasion of marked mental depression. 7. Where the varicocle prevents acceptance for either of the Government services.

There are many plans for securing the radical cure of varicocele, including castration, excision of the veins, the actual cautery, forcipressure, and ligature. The ligature is the method most commonly adopted, and has been variously modified by Ricord, Vidal, Erichsen, Wood, and

H. Lee. (These methods of treatment were then described.)

Of the efficacy of these treatments there can be no doubt, but unfortunately they have two drawbacks—the pain attending them, and a certain amount of danger. For a long time surgeons avoided as far as possible any interference with veins, and although veins are now ligatured almost as freely as arteries, *there is no doubt that diffuse thrombosis, embolism, and septic poisoning* are more liable to follow injuries of veins than of arteries. This being so, it is plainly the surgeon's duty to avoid in every possible way any irritation or disturbance of an injured vein, and it is because this principle is not sufficiently carried out that the *usual modes of treating varicocele have been attended with serious and even disastrous results.* The daily twist of Vidal's pin, and constant traction of Wood's spring, are not only painful, but opposed to the great principle that demands perfect rest to all inflamed

and injured tissues, and veins in par-
ticular, while in Lee's operation, the
presence of two hair-lip pins transfixing the
*scrotum is apt to set up œdema and inflam-
mation,* and their removal is not without
risk of *embolism.* That these are no
imaginary fears is evident from the published results of these and analogous
treatments. Gant says that the results of
the operations are "*variable,*" and include
diffuse inflammation and *sloughing of the
scrotum, suppuration of the testicle, phlebitis,
pyæmia,* and *death* ; Erichsen records *two
deaths* from the twisted suture ; Gross
had *one death* after ligature ; Sir E. Hume
had *one nearly fatal case* ; Escallier mentions *two fatal cases* of phlebitis, and
Curling speaks of *three cases of serious
results, two of which were fatal.* Some
years ago the censor of one of the chief
London hospitals *died from pyæmia after
Lee's operation. This list by no means
includes all the accidents of these treatments*
—it makes no mention of the pain suffered,

·or *of the inflammatory œdema and suppuration of the scrotum.*

It was with the hope of avoiding these complications that I was led, now more than two years ago, to try the plan of subcutaneous division of the veins by means of a platinum wire heated to a red heat by electricity. The procedure is, as you have seen, very simple. First, feel for the vas deferens and grasp the veins in front of it, and nip in the scrotum with the left thumb and forefinger ; transfix the scrotum at this spot between the duct and the veins with a narrow bistoury, and pass a needle armed with a platinum wire in the track of the knife ; then return the needle through the same apertures, but this time in front of the veins between them and the skin. Of course, if the vas happen to be in front of the veins, as was the case in that of W. C——, shown to-day, you modify the procedure a little. In this way you have the veins in a loop ·of the wire. It is better to make a puncture with a knife rather than merely to transfix with the needle, for the veins are looped up cleaner, there is not the same liability to include a portion of the skin in the noose as in the latter plan. Then attach the ends of the wire to the écraseur, and connect with the battery, using sufficient cells to cause a faint hissing noise ; one cell of Grove's battery, or at most two, is sufficient. This step must be done deliberately ; I have taken as long as five or six minutes over it. To protect the skin from burning, let some cold water trickle over it while the wire is burning its way through the veins. The after-treatment consists in perfect rest in bed for a few days, with the scrotum supported on a broad strip of strapping fixed across the front of the thighs. I have three times operated without anæsthesia, but the pain may be severe, and I prefer to have the patient under the influence of ether. After recovery from the anæsthesia there is an entire absence

of pain and this perfect freedom from
spontaneous pain continues uninterrupted
throughout the convalescence. A few
hours after the operation the knobby feel
of the varix is replaced by a soft even
swelling, which lessens and hardens, and
at the end of forty-eight hours is usually
to be felt as a hard lump, about the size
of a big marble. This is tender on pressure.
By the end of a week it has lost its tenderness, and has shrunk to three-quarters its
original size. The veins below can still
be felt full, but not compressible, the blood
in them has by that time coagulated, and
they become smaller and firmer, until ulti-
mately a small pea-like induration in front
of the vas is all that is left, and even this
may disappear, and no trace of the varix
or operation be left, as in W. S———.

I have employed this method eight
times, each time the varix has been cured,
the symptoms complained of relieved, and
no mischief to the testicle has followed.
These eight cases have shown me that there

are three things to be carefully avoided.
The first is hurry in the section of the
veins ; twice a few drops of blood have
followed the escape of the wire, but only
so little as to require nothing more than
lint or cotton-wool to be placed over the
wound ; in neither instance was there any
hæmatocele. The second is to operate
well above the tunica vaginalis, *in one of
my cases acute hydrocele was lighter, up*, it
quickly subsided under belladonna fomen-
tations. The third is burning of the skin,
leading to *a small slough ;* although there
is nothing of serious moment in this
slough, it is of course best to avoid it, and
if the skin is incised and kept cold and the
loop of wire not brought too small it can
generally be saved.

I can recommend you to practise this
operation, first, because of its entire pain-
lessness *after* the few moments of its actual
performance, and, secondly, because it fulfils
the physiological indications better than any
other I know of. My cases at present are

too few to prove by statistics *that it is less dangerous to life* than those operations I have mentioned, but they are sufficient to show that the operation is simple, effectual, and introduces no new danger, while it is obviously free from the sources of irritation common to other methods.

The section of the veins is completed at once ; there is no foreign body liable to set up inflammation left in contact with the healing veins, which are allowed to remain at perfect rest, while their seared ends are becoming permanently closed. As you are aware, the closure of an open vessel by the hot wire or iron is usually considered a particularly safe plan. There is also no interference with the skin of the scrotum, as in Lee's operation ; no compression of the scrotal vessels, no œdema.

The only other method that I should at all recommend to you is the use of the catgut ligature applied to the veins subcutaneously. I have had no experience in

it. but it has been done with success.
I think the heated wire is preferable,
because the catgut ligature is rather uncertain in its action ; it may soften very
rapidly and then fail to occlude the vessels,
or it may not soften at all, and cut its way
through the veins like an ordinary hempen
or silken thread, or remain and subsequently
light up inflammation. These accidents are
only occasional, but we should none the less
be on our guard against them, and give the
preference to a plan of treatment which is
free from them. In none of my eight cases
has any slough separated from the veins ; the
eschar formed has been absorbed by the living
tissues. I show you to-day four cases at
varying periods after the operation illus-
trating their progress.

1. W. J——, aged seventeen, a large
left varicocele, which he had noticed for
"several years," left testicle smaller than
right, complained of dragging pains in
scrotum and up to left loin. Operation

June 21st, 1879 ; left hospital June 28th.
A firm induration the size of a marble felt ;
not tender ; veins below plugged.

2. F. L——, aged twenty-four, single,
injured left testicle five years ago ; first
noticed varicocele three years ago, after
an attack of clap, since then the pain
and swelling had steadily increased in
spite of wearing a suspender. No constipation ; external piles for two years.
Operation May 28th ; left hospital June
8th. The induration is very hard, the
size of a horse bean ; veins below are
firm and shrinking.

3. W. C——, aged thirty, single, very
large left varicocele noticed suddenly in
June 1879, while bathing. Pain in scrotum
and groin had increased of late ; l testicle
smaller than right. Operation May 1st ;
left hospital May 7th ; delayed on account
of a slough of skin. Induration now
small ; veins below cannot be felt ; testicle

has regained its former size and is a little larger than right.

4. W. S——, twenty-one, a small varicocele noticed some years ; scrotum not lax ; considerable pain ; frequent seminal emissions and mental depression. Operation September 29th ; left hospital October 9th. No trace of dilated veins or of the seat of the operation to be felt. All symptoms relieved.

I should state that the italics in the foregoing quotation are mine. Mr. Gould does *not* even maintain that his operation by the galvanic écraseur is *less dangerous to life* than the other modes of operative treatment. Was any one of these four cases sufficiently severe and hopeless to warrant an operation ? Mentioning that one testicle is larger than the other proves nothing, as that is the normal state of all. Note also case 3—here the operation was performed on May 1, and patient was discharged on May 7, and shewn on July 3, so that he was under observation during two months, and such is the efficacy of an operation by the galvanic *écraseur* that we are informed that the testicle, which was smaller than the right one, not only regained its supposed original size—all in the space of about two months—but actually it "is a little larger than right." What mental myopia !

Now let us just reflect on this last word of orthodoxy in the treatment of varicocele. Mr Gould says

6

"no mischief to the testicle has followed." How does he know ? Just
look at the *dates* of his cases. In the
one of *longest* date, just *one year* has
elapsed since the operation. In this
period we have not time to see
whether there will result a withering, or a pseudo-hypertrophy. In
the third case, says Mr Gould, the
"testicle has regained its former
size and is a little larger than
right." That is to say, hyperplasia of *connective tissue* has be-
gun, and *that* testicle is probably
doomed to get very large *and useless,*
for these *enlarged* testicles are mere
masses of tissue, and no real testicles
any longer. Let us further note
the ages of these patients : 17, 24,
30, and 21, and all *single.*

Of course this able *surgeon* believes he did the right thing by these poor young men ; no man can go beyond his light, but we believe that he did them not only no real permanent service, but we maintain that to operate thus on young single men for an affection of this kind is unjustifiable. At least medicines should have been carefully and persistently tried first.

Be it remembered that patients at times *die* of operations for varicocele ; and Mr Gould himself admits that he cannot yet prove from statistics that his special operation by the galvanic *ecraseur* is less dangerous to life than other operations that he himself condemns. We admit that Mr Gould *is* a

first-class *surgeon*, but, THE BETTER
THE SURGEON, THE WORSE THE
PHYSICIAN.

This surgical treatment of varicocele may be very grand from a
surgical standpoint, but it is a bitter
commentary on the state of *medicine*
at our public Hospitals and in the
profession at large. So I proceed
with my task.

CASE OF HÆMORRHOIDS CURED WITH *Nux* AND *Sulphur*.

Some six or seven years since,
a lady, about 40 years of age, came
under my observation. She was
suffering from external piles, but
otherwise was in perfect health and
of magnificent physique. She had

taken advice on the subject of her complaint, and an operation had been determined upon, for which purpose she intended to go to her native city Dublin; but a lady friend of hers, having been admitted to her confidence, told her that the homœopaths were in the habit of treating this affection successfully with medicines. She did not expect to be cured, but thought there could be no harm in trying the homœopathic method of treatment.

An eight-weeks' course of *Nux vomica* 30, and *Sulphur* 30, resulted in a complete cure. Nothing remained of the tumour whatever. The diet was not altered, and no local application of any kind was used. The case was recent, and not severe, but yet severe enough for her to have been advised an operation.

Thousands of cases of piles may be cured with *Nux* and *Sulphur* alone ; almost any dilutions will act, but the thirtieth is more *enduring* in its effects apparently than lower ones. *Sulphur* is a grand polychrest from the crude substance upwards, but. *Sulphur* 30 is a mighty prescription. We get used to its wondrous effects, and cease to marvel thereat, just as we cease to wonder at the electric telegraph or steam locomotion.

I have repeatedly seen *Sulphur* 30 PRODUCE piles, and I once saw *Sulphur* C. cause a rather severe attack of piles. "I used to suffer from piles, but I have cured myself with *Nux* and *Sulphur*," is an oft-told tale.

The use of *Sulphur* in piles is not contained to homœopathic practice by any means, but the use of crude *Sulphur* rarely finishes a case, because its action seems to become what, in my mind, stands as *circular :* it does the good, and then goes over to the opposite action and reverses the good.

Sulphur is *the* great portal-system medicine with Rademacher in his organopathic division of abdominal complaints. His article on the subject of portal stasis is most excellent.

The diagnosis of dilatations of

the portal vein or of its tributaries
is no easy matter, as the symptoms
may be so varied. Many of those
old chronic cases of "liver" are
in reality portal congestion ; the
sufferers therefrom have generally
tried many physicians and many
medicines, and get a little relief,
but soon are as bad as ever. It is
clearly *the liver*, and yet the very
best treatment has failed. They
have often had the right remedies,
but did not take them long enough ;
in vein affections we have to deal
with a *state* that will only yield to
well followed up *coup sur coup* treatment.

Rademacher's remarks on the
diagnosis of affections of the portal-
vein system *(Erfahrungsheillehre,*

p. 290, *et seq.)* are very instructive.
He says : "The symptoms and
conditions that I have seen arise
from abdominal plethora are indeed
manifold. In first line stands
hypochondriasis, then follow giddi-
ness, visual disturbances, chronic
inflammation of the tonsils and of the
uvula, cough, asthma, hæmoptysis,
urinary troubles of various kinds ;
the so-called cold rheumatism, or
those chronic pains that many feel
in the shoulder joints ; that pain
in the heels (gallstones and hepatic
obstruction cause these same pains
in the heels), that does not prevent
walking, but makes it painful to
do so, and renders the gait stiff.
Then, less frequently, colic ; cramp
in the stomach, especially during

digestion ; sciatica ; impotence or salacity, or both. All these I have myself seen. The question is : How can we differentiate between a primitive affection of the liver, pancreas, spleen, bowels, and mesentery and plethora of the portal system ? This differentiation is not only difficult, but in many cases simply impossible."

And then he presently gives a very valuable clinical hint, viz. : the use of organ-remedies to aid the diagnosis. He says (p. 292) . . . "At times we cannot get to the bottom of these obscure cases except with the aid of *trial remedies (Probemittel)*. For instance, in some cases abdominal plethora disturbs the functions of the liver ;

then we have pain and fulness in
the right hypochondrium, the secretion of bile more or less disturbed,
a yellow dirty colour of the face,
yellow urine, difficulty of breathing,
and the like. Now if we act with
reliable remedies on the organ that
appears primarily affected, on the
liver, we either do no good at all,
or the symptoms disappear sooner
or later gradually, but the amelioration is, nevertheless, not felt by the
patient. For before you can turn
yourself round the spleen begins to
cry out, or there is pressure on the
umbilical region, or some other
discomfort crops up, seemingly
involving another organ; then, if
we have the luck to get rid of
this new affection, the liver begins

the old tune again. When we get
this wonderful hither and thither
condition, you may safely bet that
we have to do with abdominal
plethora ; provided always that no
worse disease lies hidden behind
all this, such as scirrhus."

This *organ-testing* I have found
of great importance in practice, but
it cannot be utilized unless one is
well acquainted with the organ-
remedies,—that is to say, with the
local electivity of drugs, respectively
the homœopathic specificity of seat,
which is equivalent to the organo-
pathy of Rademacher.

The periodic *orgasmus humorum*
to which those subject to hæmorrhoids are so liable is, according to
Rademacher, usually amenable to

Sulphur; sometimes it is a mixed complaint, and calls for *Sulphur* and *Sodæ nitras.*

The ancient physicians maintained that *Sulphur* is a *lung-balsam*, ; this Rademacher ridicules, but maintains that *bad coughs, and even phthisis*, may be cured with *Sulphur*, when they arise secondarily from an affection of the portal system.

THE VENOUS ZIG-ZAG LINE.

By the way, there is a pathognomonic appearance of the chest, in some cases of disturbances in the portal system, and to which I desire to call attention, viz. : We find *marked on the cutaneous surface of the chest, about corresponding* *to the costal insertions of the diaphragm, a zig-zag line of small veins.* I have never read about this, as far as I remember, but I often see it when examining patients with chest and abdominal complaints, and in my case-takings I call it the *venous zig-zag.* No doubt others observe it as often as myself. When the patients get better, this venous zig-zag becomes less and less visible.*

Before going to what I have further to say on the amenability of piles to medicinal treatment, I will just give very short notes of a case of varicocele.

---

* Dr Edward Blake has made the same observation.

CASE OF VARICOCELE.

When practising in Chester I treated a patient at the Chester and North Wales Homœopathic Dispensary for varicocele. The subject was an Irish workman of herculean stature, and who had syphilis ; after getting rid of most of the manifestations of this vile malady, I set to work at the *varicocele.* In this case *Fluoric acid* was indicated, not only on account of the dilated spermatic veins, but because of the *moist palms* and loss of hair. Indeed *Acidum fluoricuu* is no mean antisyphilitic remedy in the later manifestations, such as loss of hair, whitlows, and bone disease ;

so this was given for a number of weeks with very marked benefit, the varicocele having considerably diminished. At this stage the man ceased attending, having gone on a drinking bout, as I subsequently ascertained,

CASE OF
CHRONIC PILES WITH PROLAPSE
OF THE RECTUM.

Some three or four years since a gouty gentleman of about 50 consulted me for this distressing malady. For many years he had suffered from hæmorrhoids, with prolapse at each stool; he had been treated with various domestic remedies, and by several medical

men, both allopathic and homœopathic, and had obtained temporary
relief at various times. Besides
this he had a medicine chest of
his own, and a Domestic Vade-
Mecum, according to whose direc-
tions he was in the habit of taking
Nux, *Sulphur*, and other such well-
known remedies. He was of spare
habit, very abstemious in all respects,
and a careful liver. His bowels were
inclined to be costive, but still they
acted most days. All his organs
seemed healthy, and there was no
evidence of any disturbance in the
portal system, but he used, at times,
to pass fine sand, like brick-dust.
His going to stool was very painful,
and the act lasted a considerable
period, owing to the state of the

7

rectum ; the motion was very hard
and usually more or less streaked
with blood, and it always brought
down the bowel. After carefully
washing the part he replaced it
with more or less difficulty, and
severe pain. On account of this
unhappy state, he rarely left his
home or family, as it took him
nearly three-quarters of an hour
to get the matter over, and the
bowel washed and replaced. He
thought it came originally from
lying in the trenches in the Crimea.

In this case there was considerable hypertrophy of the rectal
mucous membrane, and also of the
subjacent connective tissue, which,
indeed, is pretty well always present
in cases of old standing.

The indications to be fulfilled were :

1. To get this tumid mass dispersed.
2. To get the hæmorrhoidal varices to contract ; and
3. To procure *easy* defecation.

Now, it may be affirmed that many physicians fail to treat such cases successfully with medicines ; they look upon them as hopeless. Granted, say they, that simple recent cases yield readily to homœopathic treatment, but these old-standing cases do not, and they must be either borne or the tumour cut away.

At first sight this seems evident, but a little thought on the subject will shew that it is not *necessarily* so.

Let us remember that we have to deal with venous stasis for the most part hypostatic, and a resultant hyperplasia of circumjacent tissue ; this goes on till a tumour is there, and *this tumid mass lies practically without the organism* to a large extent, and hence it is not reasonable to expect to affect it very radically from within, *alone*. At least that is my view of the matter, and I have, therefore, in all very severe cases of piles, made use of remedies externally—usually *Hamamelis*, sometimes *Mikania guaco*.

"Well," some reader will say, "I too have made use of *Hamamelis* externally for years, and yet bad cases for the most part will not yield to it ; I have nevertheless to have recourse to the radical operation."

To that I have several things to say. First of all as to the *mode of applying it*. A little reflection will shew that we want the thing applied for a considerable period, and my very successful plan is simply this :— Add to as much water as needful a few drops of *Hamamelis Virginica θ*—I find the ordinary homœopathic mother tincture acts better than Pond's Extract as a rule, but when the tumour is *very* painful, and active inflammation has been set up, pure Pond's Extract of *Hamamelis* may be applied as they use it in America for hurts and sprains. Then take a piece of lint of convenient size, and dip it

into the *Hamamelis* solution, and
let it become thoroughly saturated
therewith; then, on getting into bed
the patient is directed to place it
on the tumour, or just within the
anal orifice, AND LEAVE IT THERE
ALL NIGHT. This leaving it there
all night is of the greatest importance, and has helped me to cure
cases that had baffled some of
our very best men, including low
dilutionists and the very highest
dilutionists. I have noticed that
the rock on which the low-dilution
men specially are apt to strike is
the *recoil* action of their too big
doses, while the Hahnemannians, in
their laudable consistency, refuse to
sanction the local treatment.

The right diet for the hæmorrhoidal is a big chapter, and would lead me away from what I am specially pleading for in *bad cases,* viz. :—external treatment, *combined* with the internal. Neither will succeed alone, because external treatment will only aid so long as the mass cannot be thoroughly dealt with from the circulation, and local treatment is only child's play beyond a certain point, and utterly valueless to do more than influence the local mass it entirely fails to *cure* any case of itself, and is to be discontinued as soon as this can be reached well from within ; but so long as the mass is, as it were, a something outside of the body, so long must it be dealt with from the outside—a rightly chosen remedy being simultaneously administered internally. The saturated piece of lint, or other suitable material, that has lain all night at the anal orifice, should be burned, and never used a second time; it is important to insist on this, as otherwise the part may get poisoned, as it is difficult to thoroughly cleanse a *small* piece of linen.

Then, again, all aperients must be *absolutely* forbidden ; this is of prime importance, and if a patient (the case being a bad one) will not absolutely give in on this point, I invariably decline the case. There is nothing for it but this. Of course the diet must be modified accordingly. The physician who allows aperients *cannot* CURE bad piles, though he *treats* them with all the

skill of Hippocrates, Galen, Syden-
ham, and Hahnemann combined.
Why ? Because the peristaltic
action set up by the aperient acts
from above downwards, and therefore increases the hæmorrhoidal mischief mechanically, to begin with,
and then by increassing the active
congestion, and finally making the
hypostasis worse than ever.

Furthermore, it is almost of
equal importance *to forbid the
patient to go to stool until he posi-
tively cannot hold out any longer ;*
that is of course, in very severe
cases. Why ? Because hæmorrhoidal sufferers have often a knack
of *pressing* at stool as if they were
parturient; the abdominal press acts
upon the whole contents of the belly,

and thus the pressure *from above* brought to bear upon the piles will do more harm in a few moments than the best directed efforts of any physician can mend by the time another stool takes place.

It is simply not possible to cure *very severe cases* unless aperients be *totally* abandoned, and unless *all use* of the abdominal press be, for the time, given up.

"But, Doctor, I have taken aperients every day for thirty years, and I *must* have them ; and I *must* also have a motion every day, or I am so dreadfully uncomfortable, and have such a fulness in my head ; and besides, I dread the suffering of a stool if I put it off,— it is too awful."

Then, patient, go to Mr Smith and get him to do the necessary operation, for unless you obey in these points, it is simply not possible to cure such a bad case as yours with medicines ; with absolute obedience it *is* possible, and very probable.

Be it well understood that the question is now of *very severe* cases where the rectum is prolapsed and perhaps almost strangulated.

In simple cases it is often not needful to bother the patient with any change of diet whatever, but in bad oner it becomes a necessary condition of success.

I have interwoven these remarks with the narration of this case to

motive my prescription, which was
Hamamelis Virginica locally, in the
manner above described, and *Aloes
Soc.* 6, one pilule four times a day.
This was in August 1876.

Of course it will be objected
that as I used *Hamamelis* externally, and *Aloes* internally, I do
not know how much of the cura-
tive action is due to each respectively. This I grant, and the
scientific value of the prescription
is thereby lessened, no doubt.
The gentleman was away from
home at the time at the seaside
for his holidays, and this prescription was forwarded to him
by post. I had previously seen
him through several pretty bad
attacks of gout, and he had

mentioned his hæmorrhoids to me several times, but he never really consulted me about them, because, in truth, he did not believe there was any medicinal cure for them, and he did not intend undergoing any operation for them so long as he could manage to replace them, together with the bowel, after each motion. Now, however, being at the seaside, they suddenly became worse either from the sea air or his long walks, or some other cause, and being in lodgings, he missed the various little contrivances present in his bath-room at home. Moreover, they were so much worse, that walking had become most painful and barely possible. Hence he applied to me.

He did not write to me again, and remained away about six weeks. Neither did he call upon me on his return, but two or three weeks thereafter I met him accidentally, and then received his warm thanks for having relieved him of his great trouble. He informed me that he was quite well ; all the piles had disappeared, and the bowel no longer came down at stool at all ; the bowels, too, acted naturally. For fully twenty years this gentleman had almost daily suffered the horrors of a painful stool and prolapsed bowel, followed by the torture of getting it back again. Many months later I attended one of his children for fever, and learned that he continued quite well.

In the face of this experience, is any one at all astonished that I am a strong advocate for the medicinal treatment of piles, and other manifestations of the venous diathesis ? In this case I made no alteration whatever in diet, and there was no need to forbid aperients, as he had abandoned them for many years in favour of *Nux, Sulphur, Belladonna,* and *Opium,* which he knew well how to use. Indeed, alvine constipation was not an important element in this case, it was more a proctostasis.

*   *   *   *

Perhaps any further experience on the subject of the amenability of diseases of the veins to medicinal treatment may be needless, but there are two very bad cases recorded in my case-book that deserve detailed narration, because they were about as bad as such cases can well be, and they bring out another little auxiliary of mine— I mean *posture*. Minor cases I omit entirely.

ON THE IMPORTANCE OF POSTURE IN THE MEDICINAL TREATMENT OF SEVERE CASES OF PILES.

When a patient has suffered for a number of years either from continued chronic hæmorrhoids, or when he has had *attacks* of piles for a more or less lengthened period

with the well-known general *orgasmus humorum,* there comes some
fine day such a violent attack, or the
defecatory effort has been unduly
prolonged, from some cause or
other that the piles and the prolapsed bowels cannot be replaced
at all, and then *something must be
done.* There is no help for it ; the
patient lies writhing in pain, half-
doubled up, and often moans and
weeps like a child.

Now, what have we to deal
with in such cases ? Naturally,
cases differ exceedingly, and each
one must be individualized and
treated on its own merits. It is
no use confining one's ideas to the
rectum, although all the misery is
at present concentrated there, and

8

yet time presses, and patient appeals for prompt relief.

Some cases of piles depend upon a disturbance in the brain, others upon a spinal affection, especially about the *cauda equina*. Some are due to a liver complaint, and some to portal congestion ; others, again, are connected with a disturbance around the neck of the bladder, the prostate, the spermatic veins, the uterus, the ovaries ; or they may arise from chronic constipation, or be due to a really local cause in the rectum itself, mere proctostasis, or be merely a topic expression of general varicosis. Then, again, the lungs and the rectum are often in wondrous sympathy with one another. So each case has to be looked at all round, as to the other constituent organs and parts of the same economy. Then there are various nosological forms that complicate piles :—pregnancy, phthisis, gout, general plethora, cephalic congestion with threatened apoplexy (how often does apoplexy follow a wrong treatment of piles !) heart affections, and syphilis. Syphilitic hæmorrhoids are at times the most painful of any, and the pain is often an inch or two above the sphincter.

But, with *all* the varieties, there is always one prominent and distressing condition, viz.: HYPOSTASIS, in other words, *much* of the distress is due to the hypostatic congestion, and *this* it is that an operation gets rid of, and nothing else ; only, with the operation, not only is the bath emptied, but the baby has been forgotten, and poured out with it.

I have adopted the very simple plan of *raising the buttocks above the horizontal,* by means of various little mechanical contrivances improvised at the time, according to the circumstances of the patient ; two or three pillows serve the purpose. Every one is familiar with the contrivances for raising the heads of sick people ; well, I just reverse the process and raise the lower part of the trunk, and this is a great help in very severe cases, such as the following :—

In January 1880, a gentleman, about 40 years of age, residing in

London, came under my observation. He had suffered for many years from constipation and piles, with prolapse, and he had had a sorry time of it at every movement of the bowels, as the large hæmorrhoidal masses came down, together with the rectum, so that the whole resembled a big dahlia in configuration and in colour ; moreover, the constriction of the sphincter seemed so great that on my first visit, there seemed no inconsiderable danger of gangrene. His elder brother had suffered similarly, and been operated on very successfully ten or a dozen years ago, but had latterly got as bad as before the operation. My patient's sister, however, a kind-hearted capable maiden lady, who,

instead of wasting her precious life
nursing poodles, goes into the courts
and alleys of this huge city, carrying
words of comfort, and healing many
with the aid of a Homœopathic
Vade Mecum and a pocket-case of
pilules. *From her own experience (!)*
she was confident that homœopathy
could cure her brother, and this
was the more desirable as he was
very nervous and timid, and almost
fainted at the very thought of an
operation. Moreover, he is by no
means a strong man, as indeed no
one is at the end of fifteen years of
hæmorrhoidal miseries and bleeding.

On examination, I found the
usual thing : A large purple bleeding mass extending from the anus,
causing the patient such terrible

anguish that he screamed and cried. He could neither sit, lie, nor stand properly. but found least pain in lying on his side, with knees and chin considerably approximated. The size of the whole tumid mass was about that of a man's fist, and there were small ulcers on the surface, apparently suppurating excoriations.

Besides "having a liver," and being of lax fibre, he was otherwise healthy, though not strong, and of rather small stature.

I set to work in this wise :

1. I propped up the *lower* part of the body, so as to relieve the hypostasis somewhat.

2. I forbade all aperients, and any effort at going to stool : let the bowels absolutely alone.

3. He was ordered to live entirely on slops, rice and other puddings, and stewed fruit for dinner ; porridge, with simple syrup (treacle), for breakfast ; an ordinary English tea ; and gruel for supper. Beef tea occasionally ; fish every alternate day. No beef or mutton.

4. Pure Pond's Extract of *Hamamelis* constantly applied to the hæmorrhoidal tumour, and subsequently the ordinary homœopathic mother tincture *very much* diluted.

5. Internal medication.

It would be very tedious to give the ups and downs of this case and my reasons for the various remedies employed, but for the advantage of any young practitioner who may chance to read these pages, I will, nevertheless, give the bare skeleton of the treatment. Hahnemann's *Materia Medica Pura* will give him the why and the wherefore.

Jan. 27th.

Tc. Aloes 12. At first a dose every half-hour for eight doses, and then every hour.

Those who think the repetition of the dose too frequent, are reminded that the poor fellow lay writhing in agony.

28th. Considerable relief as to pain, especially after each application of the *Hamamelis*. Swelling less tense. No motion ; begs for an aperient, and permission *to try* to obtain relief of his bowels. Both absolutely refused, and *reasons given*.

29th. Easier, but otherwise no change.

Sulphur 30 every two hours, and continue the Extract.

30th. Same.

31st. Is getting frighteed about his bowels, as they have not acted.

℞ *Kali Carbonicum* 30 every two hours. (He had a cough.)

Feb. 2nd. Easier, but still no *sensible* diminution in the size of the tumour ; he is beginning to sleep better, and getting resigned

to his fate, though he is afraid of
an inflammation of the bowels from
retained fæces.

3rd. The *Kali Carb.* 30 is
continued, and *Sulphur* 30 given
in alternation with it.

Feb. 5th. The tumour is decidedly less tense, and there is now
but very little actual pain, and the
part has a much healthier hue—not
so purple. Bowels still locked,
which alarms him ; only my threat
to throw up the case keeps him
from using an aperient.

℞ *Æsculus Hippocastanum* 6 every two
hours.

9th. Notable amelioration. No
action of the bowels. Continue the
Æsculus.

12th   No action of the bowels ; renewed complaints of patient there-at.

R   *Tc. Æsculus Hippocastanum* 30 **four** times a day.

13th.   Comfortable action of the bowels, with no straining at all. Hæmorrhoidal mass withering.

Continue.

15th.   The same.

17th.   Making very rapid pro-gress ; bowels act daily, painlessly and easily, and the patient is able to put on his dressing-gown and lie on sofa. The piles are vastly improved, and the prolapse has disappeared.

Continue.

23rd. Continued progress. No change in medication. Drives out, and has white meat for dinner.

March 2nd. His condition is eminently satisfactory in all respects the bowels act beautifully every day ; of the whole anal trouble there is now scarcely anything to be seen beyond a thickening like a ring around the anus, and a large fold of skin in which the tumour had been encased.

℞ *Ferrum Phosphoricum 12x trit.* morning and afternoon.

17th. He is quite well. Nothing remains at the seat beyond a small fold of the skin like a pucker, of the size of a hazel nut, though patient is not conscious of its presence. He has now a daily motion as an act of pleasure—no piles, and no prolapse. Had not been in such a condition since his youth !

℞ *Arsenicum album* 30 twice a day, for its constitutional effect.

April 28th. Continues in all respects well. Beyond the little pucker of skin at anus everything is normal, and this exists unknown to him, and is barely noticeable, being only a shrivelled fold of the skin about the size of a horse bean ; probably the large tumour had so stretched the skin that it cannot readily contract to its primitive condition.

This case has given me very great satisfaction, and will, I trust, shew those who are faint-hearted,

whenever brought face to face with
a bad case of hæmorrhoids, that
even bad cases are perfectly amenable to homœopathic, postural, and
dietetic treatment.

At the end of the year 1876,
while practising at Birkenhead, I
was requested to visit a gentleman
residing in the neighbourhood, and
on arriving at his house was received by his wife, who told me the
following :—For many years this
gentleman then about 55 years of
age, had been a martyr to piles,
difficult defecation and prolapse of
the rectum. The bowels acted
daily, but it was in the very deed
a chirurgical operation in its actual

etymological sense, as the fæcal mass could not be dislodged without manual aid, often after a syringe, and then the prolapsed gut had to be replaced together with an enormous hæmorrhoidal mass. It must be admitted that life at such a price is dear, yet the patient had got used to it, and did not even complain. He thought it inevitable, and naturally shrank from an operation which had been often recommended to him by men of both schools and by his experienced friends. But so long as the daily manual reposition succeeded and the bleeding was not excessive, he bore it ; now, however, it had come to the usual pass, the tumour would no longer go back, simply because it was too large and *in erection,* for in severe cases of piles with prolapse the whole mass at times has the physical characters of a tense *corpus cavernosum.*

He has borne it till it could be borne no longer, and had finally decided to send for Mr B_____ to cut the whole thing off ; but his wife was afraid lest he should not get over the operation, and therefore sent for me to learn whether medicinal treatment offered any hope. I explained my views, and, after very much deliberation, the patient decided to try the medicinal treatment to please his wife ; he did not, himself, believe that medicines could touch such a severe case ; this was also, I was informed, the opinion of Mr B_____.

9

Now, it happened that this eminent surgeon, and bitter hater of our blessed homœopathy, had a very similar case just opposite in the same road, and the two families being friendly, and the cases similar, notes were compared about them. Mr B_____ operated on his patient, a lady, and I began to treat mine with medicine ; he ridiculed me openly, and by name, and I had to wait, for my victory was not yet. Of course I was not sure of succeeding ; I merely thought there was hope and promised to do my best, and my best is when I am sitting at the feet of Hahnemann.

Bland soft diet was ordered, and patient put into the right posture, such as I have already explained.

Hamamelis was applied locally, and *Aconitum*, *Belladonna*, *Nux*, *Pulsatilla*, and *Sulphur* came into play in succession. The first was on December 9th. At first we did not make much headway, and many were the doubts and fears at this period ; I myself did not then sit so firmly in the saddle as I do now.

On December 21st. *Æsculus Hippocastanum*, third centesimal trituration, every 4 hours. This was continued till recovery, and its action was most brilliant : in six weeks my patient was well enough to go to his business in Liverpool. He was not only cured of his hæmorrhoids and prolapse, but his bowels acted naturally and he felt himself stronger. It was now my turn to laugh at my chirurgical *vis-a-vis*, for his patient was *longer* recovering from the operation than mine was from medicinal treatment, and twenty-two months later she was as bad as ever, and then . . . came over to Homœopathy, and was cured.

But to return to the case under consideration : the patient remained under observation and took *Acidum fluoricum* 12 during the months of March and April ; in May and June *Natrum Sulphuricum* 3 ; and in July *Hydrastis Canadensis* 1.

The *Hamamelis* was used with occasional interruptions for six months, to get quite rid of the thickening around the anus. Then all medicine was discontinued, as he was as well as if nothing had ever been wrong with his rectum and hæmorrhoidal veins. Some of the ˋ treatment in this case was directed to the liver. This gentleman has remained well to this day, and that is more than three years since. *

Believe me, my dear allopathic brother, you may deride homœopathy till the end of your life, but it is true nevertheless.

In the end allopathy will have to kiss the cast for . . . *Magna est veritas criprævalebit.*

* Note to Second Edition : I heard from this gentleman six years later, viz., January 1886, about his daughter's health, and learn that he himself still continues well, and—strange to say—also grateful !

CASE OF CYANOSIS.

There will be no harm in giving the following practical case of Blue Disease for what it is worth :—

Morbus Cœruleus, Cyanosis, or Blue Disease. Whether this was due to a permanence of the *foramen ovale,* and thus allowing the passage of the venous blood from the right auricle to the left, or to other abnormal apertures in the septum of the auricles and ventricles of the heart, or to any other maldisposition or abnormality, or to patescence of the *ductus arteriosus,* I know not, but the subject was a young man of 25 or thereabouts. He had been a labourer in Laird's shipbuilding yards for years, but latterly had become unable for work. On my visiting him, I found him sitting propped up in a chair, his face of a deep purple blue coloration, with which we are all familiar as Cyanosis, and considerable œdema of the lower extremities, and hydrothorax; the dyspnœa was very great, and the distal ends of his fingers were clubbed in a most extraordinary degree, worse than I ever saw in the most advanced case of phthisis; a hacking cough; difficulty of speech; racking pains in all his bones and joints, so that he could neither move them nor yet remain quiet. That was just the character of the pain: *meale easier by motion.* A more perfect picture of inhuman ugliness in a human being it was never my lot to behold, and this was rendered worse by the hanging jaw and large œdematous face, and glaring bloodshot eyes. And yet his mother fondled and petted him as only mothers can ! After going over the case and learning that the cyanosis had been from his birth, and that he had only been so bad as at the present for a few weeks, I set about treating the most urgent symptoms, viz., the rheumatic pains. *Rhus toxicodendron* was given at frequent intervals. Now comes the strange part of the story : The *Rhus* not only gradually cured the rheumatism (which I expected) but it cured the œdema, the hydrothorax, the dyspnœa, *and actually lessened the general venosity very considerably,* and in the course of time even his clubbed finger ends went a little smaller. As nearly as I remember he took the *Rhus* for about three months, and he then resumed his work as labourer.

That this was a mere *fluke* on my part I need not say, neither do I now comprehend *how* the amelioration came about,—I merely narrate a most interesting clinical fact. During a period of about two years subsequent to this he used to put in an appearance at the Wirral Homœopathic Dispensary every month or two to be treated for various little colds, and the like, and then I left the neighbourhood, so I do not know what became of him, but so long as I remained at

Birkenhead he continued to work in Laird's shipyards,

I do not merely mean that this poor fellow got over his rheumatism, œdema, hydrothorax, and dyspnœa, and was then merely as blue as he had previously been, but his ordinary blueness had very materially diminished—about one-half—as his mother and the neighbours very loudly and unanimously maintained. Here the choice of *Rhus* for the *kind* of pain was strictly scientific ; its having brought about a remarkable amelioration in an old-standing case of *morbus cæruleus* is an empirical fact that I do not understand, and of which I therefore can offer no explanation.

This empirical use of *Rhus* I have since remembered with advantage.

RHUS IN THE TREATMENT OF BLUE-FACED BABIES.

I have never since met with another case of regular *morbis cœruleus*, but I have had to treat very young babies with cyanotic faces, and have here used *Rhus* 3 with striking benefit. One was an eight-month child, whose circulation was apparently not quite normal, as its face was very pale and bluish. It was not purple by any means, still everybody remarked "how peculiar, bluish, its face was." *Rhus* 3 was given, one pilule three times a day, and the beneficial effect was unmistakable, for within a very few days the face assumed a normal coloration. In several other cases in little infants in whom I had noticed a bluishness of the face, or just of the lower lips only, I have used *Rhus* with undoubted benefit : the bluishness disappeared. Quite lately a little *blonde* of two, with a *blue* lower lip, was ordered *Rhus* by me, and the blueness disappeared in a fortnight. *Quo modo ?*

HÆMORRHOIDS IN CONNECTION WITH ENGORGED SPLEEN.

A well-nourished healthy lady of fifty years of age came under observation in April 1880, complaining of the following series of symptoms . . . Pain in the left side corresponding to the region of the spleen, so bad that she cannot lie on the left side ; with this pain in the side there are two other disturbances, indicating that a kind of vascular turgescence—an *orgasmus humorued*—underlies the whole, viz. : palpitation of the heart, and piles. With these also some indigestion and a feeling as if the visceral contents of the abdomen were being pulled down.

℞ *Tc. Ceanothi Americani* 3x. ʒiv. Three drops in water three times a day.

She came from the country, so I did not see her again ; but as I asked for a report in a fortnight,

her husband wrote at the end of
that period to say that she was well
and needed no further attention.

The case of this lady rather
interested me, as some six years
previously she came under my care
for chronic headaches that seemed
climacteric ; I treated her for these
headaches, but could not make any
impression upon them, and then on
going over the various organs 1
found that the urine contained a
small quantity of albumen. This
our ordinary remedies removed in
about two months, and the headaches disappeared. About a year
later the albuminuria again returned
in a very slight degree, and with it
some cephalalgia ; both yielded at
once to the same remedies, and she

had remained well till she came with the splenalgia and hæmorrhoids. I suspect, therefore, that the old albuminuria was not due to any kidney mischief, but to venous congestion of the kidneys.

CASE OF VARICOCELE WITH VENOUS ZIGZAG.

This was a well-nourished, healthy looking gentleman of 29 years of age. He first came under observation on April 16th. He had sinned against his own body formerly, and, being happily enlightened on the subject of bodily chastity, had for years given it up, and ever since been seeking to regain his self-respect and bodily vigour,

By the way, when will fathers become sufficiently *manly* to teach lads how to become men ?

On carefully examining him, there were four points that came out :

1. There was an endocardial *bruit de souffle* most audible at the xiphoid cartilage.

2. The before-mentioned *venous zig-zag line* on the chest.

3. A left-sided varicocele these seven years ; not very large.

4. He had once had a slight attack of piles—none now.

Diagnosis : General varicosis expressed especially in the right heart, vena portæ, and spermatic veins.

TREATMENT: *Tc. Bellidis perennis* 1, ʒiv. Five drops in water three times a day.

June 2. Feels better in himself, the old feeling of *blightedness* left by the miserable habit of youth has gone. The effects of *Bellis* (common daisy) in this state, that I think of as *auto-traumatism*, is often little short of marvellous. But I cannot go into that at present. The varicocele is better; the endocardial *bruit* is less audible, he *feels* his heart comfortable now; the venous zigzag is slightly better—less distinct, but I am not so very sure about this, having only the eye to go by.

℞ *Tc. Acidi fluorici* 6, m. xxiv. Sac. lac. qs. Div. in p. æq. xxiv.

To take one powder in a little water at bedtime, and report progress in a month.

10

July 3. The varicocele is *much* smaller ; it formerly became very much more distended towards evening, especially after his having been on his feet a good deal all day, and notably *worse in hot weather ;* but now he has no inconvenience from the varicocele *even after being on foot all day in this hot weather*. The endocardial *bruit* can now be heard only with difficulty. I hear very well indeed with both ears, yet the acuity of the right one is greater than that of the left (is it so in everybody—*i.e.*, do the ears differ *normally ?*) and this quality of my hearing I make use of for differential diagnosis when using the stethoscope. Now I could formerly easily hear this bellows murmur with either ear, now I can barely hear it with the right aided by the stethoscope. By the way, we want some clinical acoumeter to aid us in coming to an apinion as to the quantitative value of endothoracic sounds for many of these bellows murmurs proceeding from the heart *do* disappear under treatment ; may be they are only hæmic but anyway we want to gauge them.

Patient is informed that in my opinion he is well, and fully fit for marriage. To this end he had sought advice. Of course, the result requires consolidating with some further medicinal treatment, but taking a drop or two of *Acidum fluoricum* 6 at bedtime does not

seriously interfere with any human
duties even if they be marital.

UNILATERAL VARICOSIS.

Apart from varicocele, which is
very commonly unilateral, one meets
in practice with a considerable number of cases of varicosis of one extremity only, and a careful diagnostic
survey generally leads to the dis-
covery of the cause. This form of
varicosis is of all the most readily
amenable to treatment, always assuming that its cause has been
accurately made out, and that said
cause can be removed. I will give
a case or two in elucidation of this :

A. A young lady, just over
twenty years of age, had very bad

varicosis of the left lower extremity, for which she had long worn an elastic appliance with much ease to the pains. Dancing and riding made the leg unbearable; and hence these pleasures, usually considered natural to her age and position, had been given up. The dancing she did not care for, as her views of the serious reality of life led her to think that rhythmic romping was unseemly, but she missed the riding very much. On my telling the Countess, her mother, that the case could, I thought, be cured by medicines, I was not believed. I found the left ovarian region occupied by a swelling of about the size of a baby's fist: it was very tender, and there was very distressing leucorrhœa of long standing. I directed my attention to curing the ovarian swelling that appeared to me to be the cause of both varicosis and leucorrhœa. It might be too tedious to detail the two years' treatment, but the result was as I foretold : the ovarian swelling very slowly disappeared, and so did, *pari passu,* the varicosis and the leucorrhœa. The elastic stocking was, of course, abandoned, and riding was resumed. Once or twice I had to treat a threatening return of the ovarian swelling, but eventually the cure proved permanent. The mother received my prognosis gracelessly, and was quite thankless for the cure ; but a physician who stands up for new theories and a heterodox practice must put up with antecedent gracelessness and subsequent thanklessness, and if he fail must bear the reproach of impurity of motive. By special grace it may not sour him.

B. An unmarried lady, of about twenty-two or twenty-three years of age, the daughter of a staff-officer, was brought to me by her mother some time since suffering from varicosis of the right leg, for which she was wearing the usual elastic stocking. Her sister had previously been operated on for ovarian disease, and on percussion and palpation a swelling in the region of the right ovary was readily

made out. She complained also
of pains in the right ovary and
right breast at this period.

The further course of the case
was just as in the last, only the
amelioration was comparatively very
quick.

I might enumerate other cases
of unilateral varicosis, but these
two exemplify all I have to say
on the subject, merely emphasiz-
ing the point that unilateralness
of effect leads me to seek unilateralness of cause, and both are
usually on the same side of the
body.

PART II.

THE first part of this little treatise is just my own clinical chat : clinical chips from my own workshop, thrown together without any attempt at classification or order, such being deemed needless. For it must obviously be much the same thing whether all the cases of hæmorrhoids come together or not, —and a dilated vein is essentially the same pathological entity whether it be portal and miscalled liver disorder, or on the legs and termed varices, or at the anus and designated piles, or round the spermatic cord and known as varicocele—it is the same thing in different localities

bearing distinctive names and resulting in varied morbid expressions,.
yet all linked together as *dilated
vein*. This idea gives the beautiful
unity in the pathology of Fletcher,
but unfortunately lost sight of but
to often in our cliniques and con-
sulting rooms : nosological names
becloud us, and in the very deed . .
*wo die Begriffe fehlen, da stellt zur
rechten Zeit ein Wort sich ein !*

Hence we consider *dilated vein*
our central idea, because we should
expect *à priori* that if *vein*-medi-
cines are a reality they will affect
the veins in any part of the body,
though, of course, local affinity or
specificity of seat will of itself render
any medicine a *vein*-remedy, and
experience teaches the truth of this.

Special organ-remedies will also be
often necessary to put right any
ᵡconsentaneous organ-disease ; and
dyscrasiæ, such as psora, syphilis,
sycosis, have the same value here
as elsewhere. It is astonishing how
many pegs there are on which
therapeutic ideas may be hung :
Paracelsus, Hahnemann, Rademacher, Fletcher, Grauvogl, Virchow,
Schüssler, Guttceit—all help.

Therefore we will consider general varicosis, varicocele, and varicose veins together, giving, however,
hæmorrhoids special consideration,
because of the peculiar anatomical
and physiological relationship of the
parts involved, but much that is
said of hæmorrhoids will apply to
other forms of dilated veins.

It is needless to say to the man
who has read and understood
Hahnemann that the accurate indi-
vidualization of each case is the
true way to wander *always*, but
generalizations and pathology must
not be neglected, for they are
most important in actual practice,
and a diagnostic survey of the
state of the various organs will be
generally necessary. At least, generalizations and pathology are tools
I cannot do without. It is a silly
proceeding to work out an elaborate
homœopathic equation in a case of
scurvy for instance, and the practitioner who understands the consti-
tutions of Grauvogl will, all other
things being equal, have more
success than he who pooh-poohs

them. Furthermore, although we certainly cannot cure all that is curable with Dr Schüssler's twelve tissue remedies, yet our knowledge of the spheres of action of these same remedies is vastly enlarged by his original way of working out his deductions.

Withal a very careful consideration of these various notions and generalizations brings us back to . . . the law of similars in its varied degrees.

It will be better to take first : *Cyanosis,* or the Blue Disease.

MORBUS CÆRULEUS.

The *Rhus*-case narrated in the first part of this treatise warrants us.

in giving *Rhus* a trial in the blue disease. Of course it cannot be expected to be a specific, but considering what it did in the case in question, and its equally undoubted beneficial effect in *lower degrees* of the same affection of which I have spoken, practical men will do well to give it a trial, as our therapeutic means in this ugly state are certainly not very numerous, even with as good a title as that now being vindicated for *Rhus*. Then it may be remembered that *Rhus* causes,— palpitation of the heart that is so violent that the body becomes moved thereby; tremor of the heart; pain in the chest as if the sternum were pressed in; dyspnœa and oppression of the chest. So we know that it affects the heart very powerfully.

For the venous state of the blood itself the Chlorate of Potassium and the Peroxide of Hydrogen have been used with undoubted benefit.

Ferrum is a most likely medicine indeed on theoretical grounds and from analogy ; the sixth trituration of the phosphate is very potent in controlling the vascular system, and it simultaneously affects the blood mass.

And referring again to

Rhus : There is also not wanting evidence of its action on the venous system, which, though not great, still is there : ":Swelling of the anal region, hæmorrhoidal tumours.'' It seems also to act pretty strongly on *muscle.*

The best study of *Rhus* with which I am acquainted is Carroll Dunham's (Lectures on Materia Medica, 1879, p. 121, *et seq.*), and this eminent man says (p. 127) : it produces an apparent *passive* con-gestion of the heart.

That *Rhus* is an important cardiac may alone be deduced from its reflected action upon the skin. It is also undoubtedly a blood-medicine.

VARICOCELE.

The remedies called for in varicose conditions of the spermatic veins will be frequently the following : *Acidum fluoricum, Pulsatilla, Silicea, Osmium, Acidum phosphoricum, Hamamelis,* and *Æsculus,* according to the symptoms.

Acidum fluoricum will be indicated when there are moist palms, pain in the left side, or a history of syphilis.

Aurum when the testicles are very small and weak, and in those suffering from mercurialism.

Silicea when there are sweaty feet, or when there is a history of a suppression of pedal perspirations, and when there are chilblains.

11

Osmium when it had been produced or aggravated by a deep, hollow, low cough, seemingly coming from low down in the body.

Acidum phosphoricum when associated with phosphaturia and pain in the testicle.

Pulsatilla will suit many cases and be specially called for in the obese and those of lax fibre and tearful mood.

Hamamelis is the prince of vein medicines, especially topically applied.

PATHOGENETIC SYMPTOM OF
Hamamelis Virginica.

I have quite lately had an opportunity of observing that *Hamamelis* is capable of producing

phlebitis. I ordered a gentleman
a lotion of *Hamamelis* to a painful
knee, resulting from a crush caused
by a neighbour's horse lurching
against it, and fixing it against the
saddle of the rider. Various applications had been previously used,
and there remained no outward and
visible sign that anything at all
ailed the knee, but it was painful
deep down. Instead of using a
few drops of the tincture diluted
with water in a compress, as I
ordered, patient applied the tincture
itself by rubbing it into the part, and
there resulted considerable swelling
of the whole region of the knee,
*and one vein swelled, stood out, and
was intensely painful to the touch.*
Thinking he was over-doing it with

the *Hamamelis*, and being, more-over, frightened, he left it off and let the inflamed and swelled part alone, and in about 24 hours it was quite well.   Here I think the *Hamamelis* caused the cellular tissue to swell and *the vein to become inflamed.*

Aconitum,   *Belladonna*,   *Nux*, *Sulphur*, and many other of our medicines will be needed in those cases in which their characteristic symptoms occur.   To give them all would be equivalent to transcribing portions of many pathogeneses, and under Hæmorrhoids this is more fully gone into.

Ferrum phosphoricum is a most powerful vein medicine, although its action on the arteries is its prime sphere ; it has cured a small aneurism in my hands (the sixth centesimal trituration), and a great indication for it is *throbbing.* It is also a beautiful hypnotic, but those who usually sleep well are often kept awake by it.

Kali chloricum is indicated in congestions, and specially in *swarthy* subjects.

Digitalis, Ceanothus, Scilla, and *Chelidonium* will sometimes obtrude themselves on general grounds, such as where the heart, spleen, liver, or kidneys are concomitantly wrong.

In the hydrogenoid constitution *Natrum sulphuricum* and *Thuja* will be thought of ; the former when the motion is so large that it pains to pass it through the rectum, and the latter when there is a history of *lues gonorrhoica,* or a neuralgia of the testicles.

Æsculus hippocastanum has cured varicocele ; disturbance in the portal system with constipation and hæmorrhoids would call for it.

Lilienthal mentions the following remedies as having been found useful in varices:—Aconitum, Aloes, Ambra, Antimonium, Arnica, Arsenicum, Belladonna, Calc. carb., Caust., china, Colocynth, Ferrum, Graphites, Hamamelis, Hepar sul., Ignatia, Kreasotum, Lachesis. Lycopodium, Nat. mur., Nux v., Platinum, Pulsatilla, Sepia, Spigelia, Sulphur, Zincum ; Ammon. mur., Acid. fluoricum, Hydrocot., Millefol., Pæon., Staph. ; Ferrum phos.

for young people. Fluoric acid for
old persons. (Homœopathic Therapeutics, 1879, p. 799.)

That *Ferrum phosphoricum* acts
Brilliantly in the old, and *Acidum
fluoricum* in the young, I can vouch
for from my own experience.

HÆMORRHOIDS.

This affection is probably as old
as mankind, and is often mentioned
in the Bible.

The name is derived from the
Greek αἱμορροΐδες, its chief symptom
being a flow of blood. Other names
are Haimorosis, Proctalgia hæmorrhoidalis, Morbus hæmorrhoidalis,
Piles, Emerods.

Ancient peoples regarded affections of the genitals and anus as

divine punishments, Thus . . . "The Lord will smite thee with the emerods" (Deut. xxviii. 27). But it is clear that many different diseases are meant under the name emerods, or hæmorrhoids, such as tumours, the morbus ficarius, and the endless ills of the *pathici* (Hippocrates ; Aristotle ; Rosenbaum's *Geschichte der Lustseuche*).

The piles do not usually get well of themselves.

Heart affections; imperfect æration of the blood ; liver affections ; congestions in the portal system of veins ; enlarged spleen ; abdominal tumours ; great accumulation of fat in the omentum, or of fæces in the intestines ; in fact, anything that disturbs the reflux of blood to the right heart, vena cava inferior, vena portæ, tends to hypostatic hyperæmia of the hæmorrhoidal veins. The successful treatment of piles involves an accurate appreciation of the topography and of the anatomical relations from the midriff to the pelvic outlet as first groundwork, and then a consideration of the etiology of each case.

I cannot enter upon such an interminable path in this little tract, as I merely put in a plea for the exclusively medicinal treatment of dilated veins by what name soever they may be nosologically baptized. The bulk of my own knowledge on the subject has already been given, and I now bring together from various sources the remedies most frequently called for, together with, more or less accepted, indications for the same.

REMEDIES FOUND USEFUL IN THE TREATMENT OF DILATED VEINS, PARTICULARLY OF *Hæmorrhoids*.

Besides Gilchrist, Hughes, Hale, and Lilienthal, I have culled from a very able article on this subject in the Transactions of the Homœo- pathic Medical Society of the State Pennsylvania, vol. II. The authors are the Alleghany County Homœo- pathic Medical Society, and the names of the special contributors are Drs Childs, Martin, Caruthers, and Edmundson, the last-named of whom says . . . "For the latest and most successful remedies used

by the old school for the treatment
of hæmorrhoids, we refer you to
Naphey's *'Therapeutics,'* where a
very full and complete *résumé* will
be found ; many of them you will
recognise as well-known homœopathic remedies." Well, we had
already previously gone to Naphey's
"Modern Medical Therapeutics,"
sixth edition, 1879, but did not find
anything of the kind, and on again
hunting therein we do not find even
the words piles, hæmorrhoids, varices, varicosis, or varicocele, any-
where. So, Probably, there must
be another Naphey's Therapeutics.

ACONITUM NAPELLUS.—When a
febrile movement accompanies the
piles, with dry skin and cephalic

congestion. It is not often called for in practice in this affection, but in plethoric subjects in whom there is determination of blood to the head, a prompt use of this remedy may avert apoplexy. When this is done, see to your patient's diet.

ACIDUM ACETICUM.—Profuse hæmorrhoidal bleeding ; hæmorrhage from bowels after checked metrorrhagia ; constipation ; malignant disease of rectum.

ÆSCULUS GLABRA.—The greater pathogenic power of this remedy should lead us to think of it especially when there is a paretic state of the legs, and the *cauda equina* is disordered. Carrying the nut on the person is said to cure piles, but I will not vouch for it.

ÆSCULUS HIPPOCASTANUM.—Dr
Hale is of opinion that the *central
point of action* of this drug lies in
the *liver and portal system.* It is
decidedly one of our most powerful
remedies for piles *and constipation.*
My own notion of its applicability
points to those cases in which there
are liver, portal, rectal, and spinal
indications for its use. Hale says
the *absence of actual constipation*
differentiates between this and other
pile remedies : to this I cannot
assent, my own pretty extensive experience with it leads me to say with
Dr Hughes that it *is* indicated in
constipation, and that very strongly.
That it is a great rectal remedy
is undoubted. Dr Hart's special
indication for it is *throbbing in the*

abdominal and pelvic cavities. Lilienthal puts the following symptoms
thus : DULL BACK-ACHE, PURPLE
HÆMORRHOIDS. Sensation as if
sticks, splinters, gravel were in the
rectum are said to be characteristic
of it.

ALOES.—Protruding piles, with
constant bearing down sensation
and prolapse of the bowel ; paralysis
of the sphincter ani.

Aloes stood of old in *evil* repute
in hæmorrhoidal affections ; thus in
Nathanael Sforzia's NEUES ARTZ-
NEYBUCH (Basel, 1684) we read, p.
34,—*Alle purgierende Sachen, son-
derlich von* ALOE, *alle gesalzenen und
gewürtzten Sachen seynd schädlich*
(in piles). So that with our law to
lead we know how to use Aloes.

How is it Sforzia was so enlightened ?
He was in his day *heterodox !*

ALUMINA.—Hæmorrhoids worse
in the evening ; better after night's
rest ; clots of blood pass from anus ;
stools hard and knotty like sheep's
dung.

AMBRA GRISEA.—Itching, smarting, and stinging at the anus ;
increased secretion of urine, much
more than the fluid drunk. *Worse*
in the evening ; also when lying in
a warm place, and on awakening.
Better from slow motion in the
open air, and when lying or pressing upon the painful part. Presence
of cholesterine in the fæces.

AMMONIUM CARB. — HÆMOR-
RHOIDS PROTRUDE, INDEPENDENT
OF STOOL.

AMMONIUM MUR.—Hæmorrhoids sore and smarting after suppressed whites ; hard, crumbling stools, requiring great effort to expel them ; bleeding from the rectum, with lancinating pains in perinæum, especially evenings ; stinging and itching in rectum before and during a stool ; the piles surrounded by inflamed pustules.

ANACARDIUM.—Lilienthal says : Internal piles, especially if fissured ; painful hæmorrhoidal tumours ; frequent profuse hæmorrhage when at stool ; great and urgent desire for stool, but the rectum seems powerless, with sensation as if plugged up ; great hypochondriasis.

ANTIMONIUM CRUDUM.—Copious hæmorrhoidal hæmorrhage accom-

panying a stool of solid fæcal matter;
MUCOUS PILES ; pricking burning ;
continuous mucous discharge, stain-
ing yellow ; sometimes oozing away
of an ichorous discharge; feeling of
soreness in the rectum as if an ulcer
had been torn open.

APIS.—When there is much
burning and excessive œdema of
the parts.

ARNICA MONTANA.—Blind hæ-
morrhoids, with painful pressure in
rectum, constipation and tenesmus ;
worse when standing and from cold
things. In prolapse from over-
straining at stool and from violent
riding.

ARSENICUM ALBUM.—Hæmor-
rhoids with stitching pain when
walking or standing, not when at

12

stool, with burning pain ; burning
and soreness in rectum and anus ;
rectum is pushed out spasmodically
with great pain, and remains pro-
truded after hæmorrhage from
rectum ; BURNING IN ALL THE VEINS,
restlessness and great debility,
worse at night and from cold,
better from warmth ; HÆMORRHOIDS
OF DRUNKARDS.

AURUM.—My own use of this
polychrest in piles has been con-
fined to syphilitic subjects aggravated by mercurial symptoms. I
should consider it especially called
for in the *aged* and *in pining* youth-
ful subjects.

BADIAGA.—I have put down the
river-sponge as an anti-hæmor-
rhoidal remedy, because Hering

says it is useful in the complaints of adults who had manifestations of scrofula in their youth, and because it has a reputation in Russia for the cure of piles. Now there is a class of persons who are strumous and hæmorrhoidal, and hence it may be worth remembering, especially when the lung or heart symptoms of Badiaga are present.

BELLADONNA.—Bleeding piles ; spasmodic constriction of sphincter ani ; violent pains in small of back as if it would break ; piles so sensitive that the patient has to lie with the nates separated ; scanty red urine ; congestion of blood to head ; red, hot face ; thirst and restlessness.

BERBERIS VULGARIS.—Hæmor-rhoids with itching and burning, particularly after stool, which is often hard and covered with blood ; soreness in the anus, with burning pain when touched, and great sensitiveness when sitting ; hard stool like sheep's dung, passed only after much straining ; constant pulsating stitches in sacrum ; fretful and weary of life.

BRYONIA ALBA.—Hard, tough stool, with protrusion of the rectum ; long-lasting burning in the rectum after hard stool ; sharp burning pain in the rectum with soft stool ; white and turbid urine ; sensation of constriction in the urethra when urinating. *Worse* in the morning, also from motion and from heat.

Better while lying down, or on getting warm in bed.

CACTUS GRAND.—Constipation as from hæmorrhoidal congestion ; swollen varices outside the anus, causing great pain ; itching of anus, pricking in the anus, as from sharp pins, ceasing from slight friction ; copious hæmorrhage from anus, which soon ceases.

CALCAREA CARBONICA.—Hæmorrhoids protruding, painful when walking, better when sitting, causing pain during stool ; great irritability of the anus, even a loose stool is painful ; frequent and copious bleeding of the piles, or for suppression of habitual bleeding (after sulphur). Perspires a good deal in the head, especially at night. The Calcarea subject is light haired.

CAPSICUM.—Piles having swollen ; itching, throbbing, with sore feeling in anus ; the tumours are very large, with discharge of blood or bloody mucus from the rectum ; blind piles with mucous discharge ; suppressed hæmorrhoidal flow, causing melancholy ; lack of reactive force, especially with fat people who are easily exhausted.

CARBO VEG.—Discharge of an acrid, corrosive, viscid humor from the anus, causing much itching and some smarting ; oozing of moisture from the perinæum, with soreness and much itching ; protruding large bluish varices, suppurating and offensive, with burning pains in the anus, stitching pains in the small of the back, burning and tearing in the limbs ; constipation, with burning stools and discharge of blood ; frequent determination of blood to the head, flatulence, slow action of the bowels ; epistaxis ; dysuria ; especially called for in debauched, used-up subjects and in profound adynamia.

CHAMOMILLA.—Bleeding piles, with compressive pain in the abdomen, frequent urging to stool ; occasional burning and corrosive diarrhœic stools ;. tearing pain in the small of the back, especially at night ; painful- and ulcerated rha. gades of the anus.

COLLINSONIA CANADENSIS.—Dr Hale believes that this remedy

has the power of contracting the
branches of the portal vein—indeed,
he inclines to believe that it has
this action on all the bloodvessels
and even on the heart. It is in common use in America as a vulnerary.
It claims a careful study and comes
into very frequent use in general
varicosis, and any of its varieties,
such as hæmorrhoids, varices, or
varicocele. And if Hale's view of
its action is right, those cases of
dilated *right* heart, passive portal congestion, with hæmorrhoids,
would be its triune sphere, and here-
by there is always constipation and
the cases are chronic and obstinate.

DIOSCOREA VILLOSA.—Dr Burt
got hæmorrhoids and yellow, thin,
bilious stools with prolapse of the

rectum, when he was proving the colic root. In another a hæmorrhoidal tumour of nearly four years' standing disappeared while proving it. Its reputation in enteralgia is now well established. Acute painful varicocele from excess in venery, or long-lasting unsatisfied desire, will make us think of *Dioscorea* or Dioscorein. *Dioscorea* is a powerful cardiac, and has cured a case of *angina pectoris* in the hands of Dr Skinner.

FERRUM.—Piles, copious bleeding or ichorous oozing tearing pains with itching and gnawing; costiveness, stool hard and difficult, followed by back-ache. We heartily endorse Schüssler's recommendation of the *phosphate,* and that in the

sixth centesimal trituration, but very
irritable subjects must not take it
at night, as it is very apt to keep
such awake. It comes in specially
after other rectal remedies have
done their work, to consolidate the
cure by reason of its profound action
on the whole systemic circulatory
apparatus.

GRAPHITES.—Piles with pain on
sitting down or on taking a wide
step, as if split with a knife, also
violent itching and very sore to the
touch ; burning rhagades at the
anus ; large hæmorrhoidal tumour,
protrusion of the rectum, without
urging to stool, as if the anus was
lame ; fissure of the anus, sharp
cutting pain during stool, followed

by constriction and aching for several hours, worse at night; chronic constipation, with hardness in hepatic region; moist humid eruption on scalp and behind ears; watery leucorrhœa at the times of menstruation; piles, accompanied by dizziness.

HAMAMELIS VIRGINICA.—The use of this remedy is somewhat empirical, but its power over hæmorrhoids and other venous sticlis such that it stands *facile princeps* at the head of them all. The stasis, its introduction into our practice is thus given: Mr Pond brought out his Extract of Hamamelis as a remedy for piles. Dr Constantine Hering was Mr Pond's family physician, and was induced by the latter to try its efficacy in some diseases, particularly in painful bleeding piles. But its virtues as a pile medicine were well known to the aborigines of North America, and the earlier settlers got their knowledge of it from them. Speaking of it in a letter to Hering, in 1853, Dr Okie says : "I next made use of Hamamelis in a number of cases of painful and bleeding piles. Those cases in which it has proved most beneficial in my hands are characterized by runing soreness, fulness, and at times rawness of the anus ; in the back a weakness or weariness, or as the patients graphically express it "Doctor, my back feels as if it would break off.' "

It is our best topic in all forms. of dilated veins. Almost all Americans *en voyage* seem to carry Extract of Hamamelis with them.

HYDRASTIS.—This plant has a reputation for many things. Undoubtedly it is a great polychrest. I should think of it for hæmorrhoids with jaundice and constipation, some other Hydrastis *symptoms* being present. I have known it *cause* balanitis and yellow balanorrhœa, with such a strong-smelling discharge that the unintentional prover had to keep away from society for several days, and so profuse that he fastened a piece of linen inside of his. shirt to help to absorb the discharge, and nevertheless his trousers were spoiled by the flux. The discharge

was very yellow, and after it had
lasted three days there was phimosis,
and on my forcing the prepuce back
it cracked in three places and bled.
There had previously been nothing
whatever wrong with the parts,
and from my knowledge of the
gentleman and a very careful ocular
examination of the parts, I can say
that there was no urethritis or
urethral flux, and no chancre or
chancroid, and there had been no
coition of any kind at this time. At
the height of the affection one of
the inguinal glands became painful
and swelled ; it all passed off in a
week with no treatment but cleanli-
ness. He had taken it about a
week, some six or eight *very* yellow
pilules a day, evidently θ or 1^x, and

"for a stitch in the liver and dirty tongue." To the best of my knowledge and belief the whole series of phenomena were pathogenetic.

IGNATIA AMARA.—SUDDEN SHARP STITCHES IN RECTUM, SHOOTING UP-WARD INTO THE BODY; evacuation of fæces difficult, because of seeming inactivity of rectum, every violent effort to expel them may produce prolapsus ani ; after stool frequent spasmodic constriction of the anus ; recurring pains in the anus, compounded of soreness, spasmodic constriction, and pressure ; moderate effort at stool causes prolapsus ani ; bleeding during and after stool ; fissures of anus ; hæmorrhage and pain are worse when the stools are loose.

KALI CARBONICUM.—Passage of fæces difficult owing to their bulk ; sensation as if the anus would be fissured ; stinging, burning, tearing, itching, screwing pain, followed even a natural stool, setting the patient nearly crazy and depriving him of sleep ; the tumours swell and bleed much ; riding on horseback ameliorates the pain for the time being ; hæmorrhoids complicating *fistula in ano,* especially in the *poitrinaires.*

KALI SULPHURICUM.—Hæmorrhoids with catarrh of stomach, and tongue coated with yellow mucus ; sensation of faintness in the stomach, and dull feeling in the head, fearing to lose her senses.

LACHESIS.—Piles PROTRUDING
AND STRANGULATED, or with stitches
upward at each cough or sneeze ;
sensation as of a plug in the anus ;
rectum prolapsed or tumefied ; ham-
mering, beating in the rectum ; worse
at the climaxis, or with drunkards.

LYCOPODIUM CLAVATUM.—Varices
protrude, painful when sitting ; discharge of blood, even with soft stool ;
itching eruption at the anus, painful to touch ; itching and tension
at the anus in the evening in bed ;
continued burning or stitching pain
in the rectum ; constipation ; ineffectual urging from the contraction
of the sphincter ani ; flatulence ;
hæmaturia ; pain in the sacral region, extending to the thighs, worse
rising from a seat. Lycopodium

13

has undoubtedly cured aneurisms of small calibre ; it lessened one in my hands while I was House-Surgeon at the Hardman St. Homœopathic Dispensary, in Liverpool. Hence its power over *blood-vessels* must be admitted.

MERCURIUS.—LARGE BLEEDING VARICES WHICH SUPPURATE;hæmorrhage after micturition ; hæmaturia; with violent frequent urging to urinate ; prolapsus recti after stool ; rectum black and bleeding ; pain in sacrum, as after lying on a hard couch, great weakness, with ebullition and trembling from the least exertion.

CYANURET OF MERCURY.—I have used this remedy in diphtheria with very satisfactory results, and hence it constitutes a part of my usual drug choice. The enormous activity of all the combinations of the metals with hydrocyanic acid leads us naturally to expect great things from the Cyanide of Mercury. It causes phlebitis and varicosis ; it has a grand future. The sixth centesimal dilution is the lowest I ever use of this deadly drug—in this strength it may be given to the tenderest babies.

German homœopathic practitioners speak highly of *Acidum hydrocyanicum* in *varicose* ulcers.

MURIATIC ACID.—Piles, suddenly, IN CHILDREN ; the hæmorrhoidal tumours are inflamed, swollen, bluish, with swelling of anal region, sore pains, violent stitches, and great sensitiveness to contact, even of the sheets ; prolapsus recti while urinating.

NITRIC ACID.— Long-lasting cutting pain in rectum after loose stool, with hæmorrhoidal troubles ; old pendulous hæmorrhoids, that cease to bleed, but become painful to the touch, especially in warm weather; HÆMORRHAGE BRIGHT RED, NOT CLOTTED, faint from least motion, bleed after every stool ; spasmodic tearing during stool from fissures in rectum ; HÆMATURIA, shuddering along the spine during micturition, and urging afterwards.

NUX VOMICA.—Blind, or bleeding piles, irregular piles ; stitching, burning or itching of the anus; stitches and shocks in the small of the back, with bruised pains so that the patient is unable to raise himself; constipation, with frequent ineffectual urging to stool, and with sensation as if the anus were closed and constricted; frequent rush of blood to the head or abdomen, with distension of the epigastrium and hypochondria; hæmaturia from suppressed hæmorrhoidal flow, or menses; ischuria, suppression of urine; backache, must sit up in bed.

PETROLEUM.—Piles and fissures at the anus, great itching; scurf on borders of anus; stool insufficient, difficult, hard, in lumps.

182 *The Medicinal Treatment*

PHOSPHORUS. — Constipation, small-shaped, hard stool, and expelled with great difficulty ; discharges of blood from the rectum, also during stool ; spasm in the rectum ; paralysis of the lower intestines and of the sphincter ani ; discharge of mucus out of the gaping anus ; stinging or itching at the anus ; the piles bleed easily ; increased secretion of pale, watery urine ; involuntary discharge of urine. *Worse* in the evening and at night, also when lying on the back or left side. *Better* when lying on the right side, from rubbing and after sleeping.

PODOPHYLLUM.—This is a remedy that I, myself, have used but very little, for the very good reason, that of late years a veritable podophyllomania has raged in this country, and almost all patients with anything wrong between liver and rectum have taken it on their own account. This regrettable abuse of a potent remedy must not deter us from bearing it in mind in suitable cases. Hale says : *"Hæmorrhoidal affections* are admirably under the control of Podophyllum. The specific affinity which this drug has for the liver, portal system, and rectum, as shown in the pathogenesis, enables it to cause hæmorrhoids from portal congestion, chronic hepatic affections, and primary irritation, congestion and even inflammation of the veins, and mucous membrane of the rectum. It will be found useful in external piles, for those which bleed and those which do not. The *sensations* it causes in the rectum, anus, and hæmorrhoidal tumours are similar to the effects of *Aloes*, of which it is a congener."

Morning aggravation is characteristic of podophyllum.

PULSATILLA NIGRICANS.—Painful protruding piles, with itching and sticking pains and soreness.

RHUS TOX.—Fissures of the anus, with periodical profuse bleeding from the anus; sore piles, protruding after stool, drawing in the back from above downwards, pains in the small of the back as if bruised, when keeping quiet; frequent urging to urinate day and night, with increased secretion; sore blind hæmorrhoids, protruding after stool, with pressing in the rectum, as if everything would come out. Worse at night, from cold, pressure, or rest.

SILICEA.—HÆMORRHOIDS IN-TENSELY PAINFUL, boring cramping sensation from the anus up the rectum and towards the testicles; protrude during stool; become in-carcerated. and suppurate; piles protrude with the stool, and dis-charge bloody mucus; can only be returned with difficulty; fistula at anus, with chest symptoms, aching, beating, throbbing, in lumbo-sacral region : anus is constantly damp.

SULPHUR.—Hæmorrhoids blind or bleeding, blood dark, with violent bearing-down from small of back towards the anus : lancinating pain

from anus upwards, especially after
stool ; suppressed hæmorrhoids, with
colic, palpitation, congestion of lungs;
back feels stiff as if bruised ; anal
region swollen, with sore, stitching
pains ; considerable quantity of
blood passed with soft easy stool ;
PAINLESS PILES ; bleeding, burning,
and frequent protrusion of the
hæmorrhoidal tumours ; weak digestion, dysuria.

VALERIANATE OF ZINC.—Dr
Dradwick noticed the fact that in
a considerable number of patients
troubled with piles, and who were
taking Valerianate of Zinc for other
troubles, the hæmorrhoids have,
with few exceptions, been relieved.
In cases of neuralgia, prosopalgia,
spinal neuralgia, and proctalgia, to-

gether with hæmorrhoids, we may be glad to remember this happy union of valerian and zinc.

VERATRUM ALBUM.— Hæmorrhoids, with disease of lungs, or pleura ; painless discharge of masses of blood in clots, with sinking feeling ; bruised feeling in sacral region. (Lilienthal.)

ZINCUM.—Constipation , stool hard and dry, inefficient, only expelled by hard pressing ; sensation of soreness, and violent itching at the anus ; tingling at the anus, as if from ascarides ; violent desire to urinate ; retention of urine when beginning to urinate. *Worse* in the afternoon and in the evening, also when in a warm room. *Better* in the open air.

CONCLUSION.

IN the First Part of this little treatise I give my own experience, and thus offered some evidence of the curability of vein affections by medicines ; I am by no means alone on this ground ; hundreds of homœopathic physicians were on it before me, and I trust, therefore, no one will suppose that I claim to have *originated* the notion of contracting dilated veins by medicines. Many of my medical friends are fond of the Surgery of the Veins ; I prefer medicine, and these pages are meant to give the grounds of my faith : for me these grounds are sufficient : what they may be for you, critical reader, I know not. If you should prefer steel, either cold or hot, well, *de gustibus non est disputandum.*

The Second Part is, for the most part, not my own, but is culled from numerous systematic and pharmacological works, and contains, I trust, all that will be needed to test the question of the curability of varices by medicines.

PUBLISHERS' NOTE

With a view to make the work more easily referable, an index has been added by the Publishers.

INDEX TO REMEDIES